David Rimmer

Films & Tapes 1967–1993

A Fraser Elliott Foundation Canadian Contemporary Exhibition

David Rimmer

Films & Tapes 1967–1993

Art Gallery of Ontario

Musée des beaux-arts de l'Ontario

Toronto

Canadian Cataloguing in Publication Data

Main entry under title:

David Rimmer : films 1967–1993

Includes bibliographical references.

ISBN 1-895235-40-5

1. Rimmer, David, 1942–   – Criticism and interpretation. I. Art Gallery of Ontario

PN1998.3.R5D3 1993   791.43'023'092   C93-095155-7

The Art Gallery of Ontario is funded by the people of Ontario

through the Ministry of Culture, Tourism and Recreation.

Additional operating support is received from the Municipality

of Metropolitan Toronto, Communications Canada, and

The Canada Council.

This exhibition is organized and circulated by the Art Gallery

of Ontario with the financial assistance of The Fraser Elliott

Foundation, Exhibition Assistance Program of The Canada Council,

and the Canadian Filmmakers Distribution Centre.

Contents

Preface

Following the pioneering work of Michael Snow, Joyce Wieland, and others in the early 1960s, a second generation of film artists emerged in Canada in the late 1960s. Vancouver formed one of the crucial centres with such artists as Gerry Gilbert, Al Razutis, Sam Perry, and Keith Rodan. The work of David Rimmer, however, has perhaps played the biggest role in defining Canadian film and video art in this period.

Rimmer worked in New York City from 1971 to 1974, where he engaged a variety of media including video, dance, performance, installation, and film, often with vanguard artists like Yvonne Rainer. In retrospect, however, it is the small body of poetic film work produced in 1969 and 1970 in Vancouver and the *Canadian Pacific* films from the mid 1970s which established Rimmer's reputation internationally as one of Canada's most compelling film artists. What this volume aims to establish, however, is that Rimmer is a film artist whose richest and most challenging work has been created, and continues to be created, since 1984. This work has also been the most eclectic formally, with Rimmer engaging in critically reprocessing media imagery (e.g., *As Seen on TV*), *cinéma verité* travelogues (e.g., *Black Cat White Cat It's a Good Cat if It Catches the Mouse*), dance videos (e.g., *Roadshow*), and a tour de force of montage (*Beaubourg Boogie Woogie*). Furthermore, while Rimmer has worked in video for almost as long as he has worked in film, his projects since 1989 have demonstrated an increasing interest in film/video hybrid projects. Few artists in the world – and no artist in Canada – have embraced both media simultaneously with as much confidence and facility as Rimmer. Finally, with the work from *Bricolage* (1984) onwards, Rimmer engages in a rigorous exploration of issues especially pertinent to contemporary art: the representation of gender, spatial and temporal dislocation, and notions of framing and containment.

This volume accompanies a retrospective of Rimmer's films and videotapes produced since 1984, screened on a rotating basis at the Art Gallery of Ontario between 19 October and 28 November 1993, as well as screenings of films by Rimmer's colleagues in both Canada and the United States who share his formal and thematic concerns. Following the Art Gallery of Ontario's exhibition, a retrospective of all of Rimmer's film and video work from 1967 to the present will tour numerous Canadian and American venues.

I am indebted to David Rimmer for his cooperation at every stage of the exhibition and catalogue. Professor Catherine Russell of Concordia University is to be thanked for her enthusiastic commitment to creating virtually the first scholarly overview of an artist whose work has not hitherto received the critical attention it deserves. Kathryn Elder, Moving Image Librarian at York University, is to be thanked for her painstaking research on the critical literature on Rimmer's work, most of it published in obscure sources, hitherto beyond the immediate reach of film enthusiasts. Dawn Caswell compiled the filmography, videography, and chronology. Kathryn MacKay identified and prepared frame enlargements for the publication.

We owe our appreciation to Fraser Elliott and the late Betty Ann Elliott for their support of contemporary Canadian exhibitions such as these.

The exhibition, catalogue, and tour have also been generously supported by the Canada Council. The Canadian Filmmakers' Distribution Centre assisted the Gallery with the presentation of work contextualizing Rimmer's career.

Jim Shedden
Assistant Curator, Film and Video
Art Gallery of Ontario

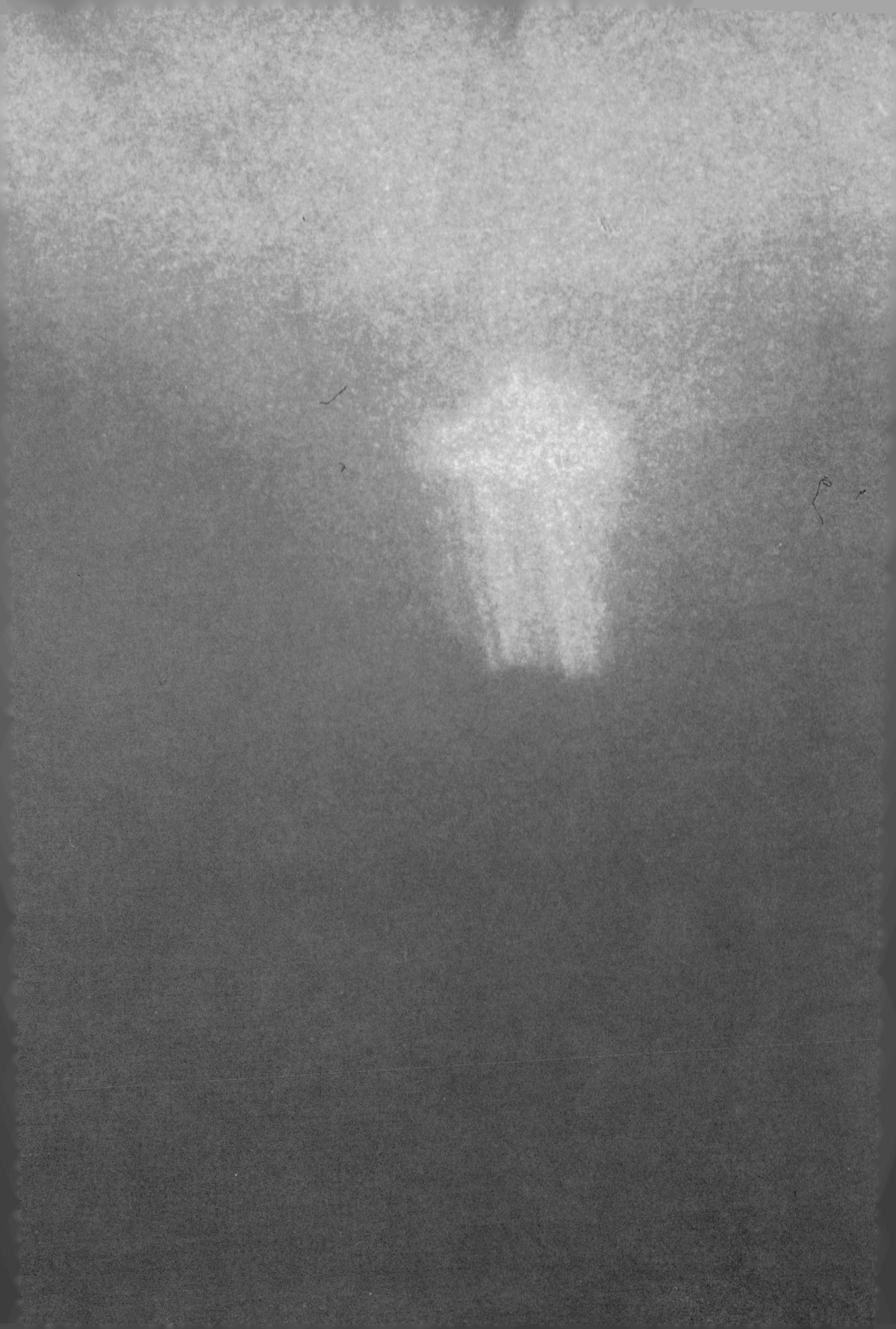

Chronology

1942   Born in Vancouver

1963–67   Attends University of British Columbia, Vancouver

1968   Begins MA in English at Simon Fraser University, Burnaby

1968–69   Negative cutter at CBC, Vancouver

1968–71   Produces numerous tapes both alone and in collaboration with other artists through Intermedia Film Cooperative, Vancouver

1969–70   Film editor at CBC, Vancouver

1971   Performs with Yvonne Rainer's dance company, New York City

1971–74   Works in New York City under two Canada Council grants; freelance cameraman and editor, New York City

1971–73   Works with video artists Rudy Stern and John Reilly at Global Village, New York City

1974–79   Sessional film and video instructor and studio techniques foundation course instructor, Department of Fine Arts, University of British Columbia, Vancouver

1977   Replacement film instructor, Vancouver School of Art, Vancouver

1979–84   Sessional film and video instructor, Simon Fraser University, Burnaby

1983   Visiting artist, San Francisco Art Institute, San Francisco

1983   Participates in Dance for the Electronic Age, a ten-day workshop in dance and video Toronto

1984   Awarded First Prize Performance – Company Category, Dance on Camera Film Festival, New York City; creates a promo tape for Karen Jamieson Dance Company

1984–present.   Video instructor, Emily Carr College of Art and Design, Vancouver

Selected Exhibitions and Screenings

1969   Thirty-monitor video installation, Vancouver Art Gallery, Vancouver

1970   Intermedia event involving poets, film, and light, Edmonton Art Gallery, Edmonton;
Intermedia Spring Show, film installation and environment design for dance
performance, Vancouver Art Gallery, Vancouver;
Kinetic Light, film installation, Art Gallery of Greater Victoria, Victoria

1975   *Show of Numbers*, video installation, holography, and sculpture, Vancouver
Art Gallery, Vancouver

1978   Two-screen film installation, Winnipeg Art Gallery, Winnipeg

1979   *13 Cameras*, photography, Vancouver Art Gallery, Vancouver;
13 Cameras, photography, National Film Board Still Photo Gallery, Ottawa

1980   *David Rimmer Films*, films and sculpture, Vancouver Art Gallery, Vancouver

1983   *Vancouver: Art and Artists 1931–1983*, films, Vancouver Art Gallery, Vancouver

1986   *As Seen on TV*, video installation, Charles Scott Gallery, Vancouver

1987   Video installation, Charles Scott Gallery, Vancouver

1988   Video installation, Charles Scott Gallery, Vancouver; film screening, Beijing Film
Academy, Beijing

1989   Film screenings: International Experimental Film Congress, Toronto; Toronto
Festival of Festivals, Toronto; Vancouver International Film Festival, Vancouver;
Museum of Modern Art, New York City

1990   Film screening, Kino Arsenal, Berlin

1991   Film screening, Béla Bálázs Studio, Budapest

1992   Film screenings: Moscow Film Union, Moscow; Centre Pompidou, Paris (France)

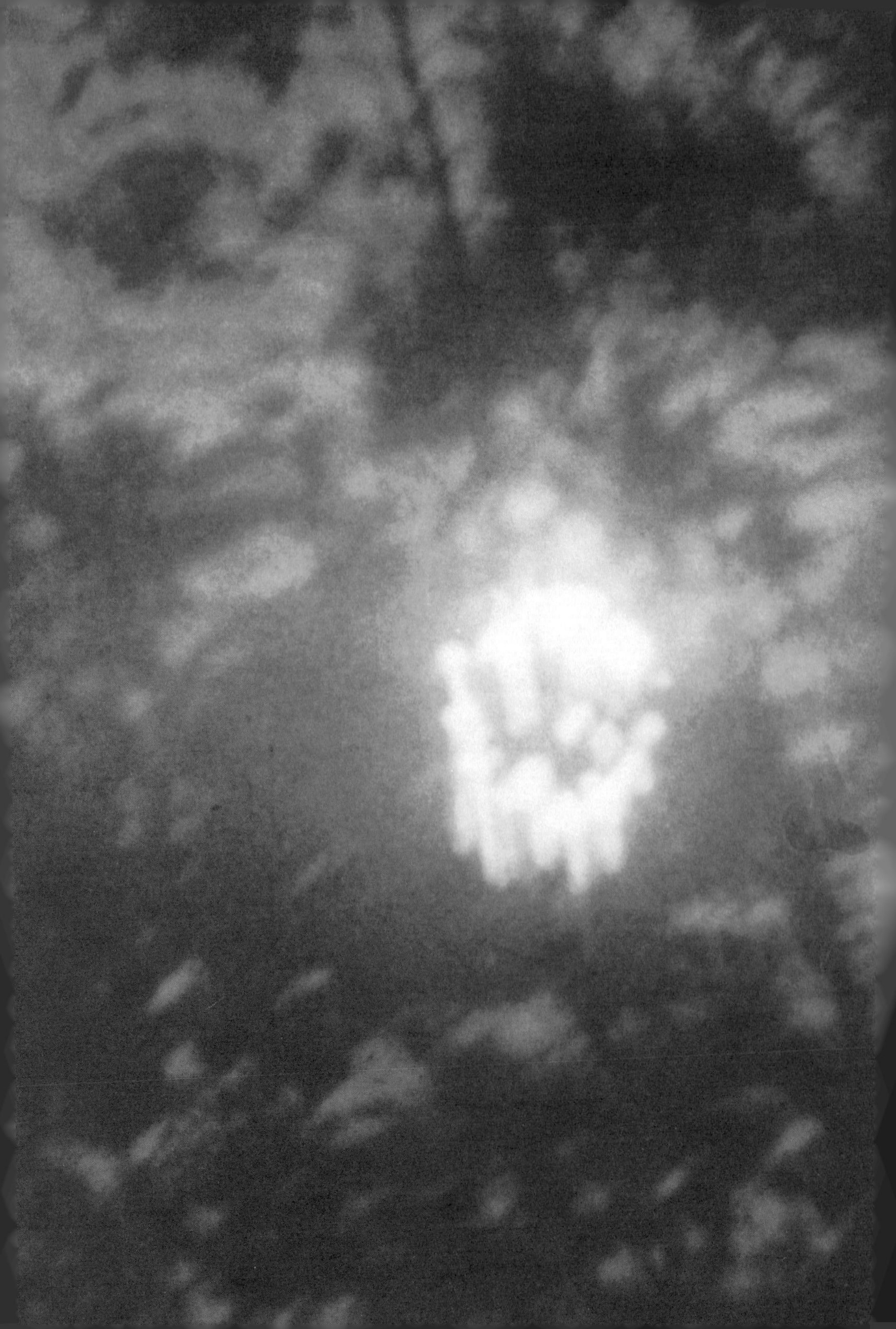

David Rimmer:
Twilight in the Image Bank

Catherine Russell

Introduction: Experiment Results

The avant-garde dies in discourse, as discourse, perhaps all discourse on
the avant-garde is its death; it was never distinct from its death, indeed
death was always its most abiding force; it sought death in order to reflect
it better, to become the reflection of a reflection, to conclude nothing but
to go on articulating its exhaustion. What we witness today is not a termi-
nus, since advanced art appears in ever greater profusion, but the becom-
ing-(death)-discourse of the avant-garde within an economy in which
nothing is more vital than death.[1]

On 1 June 1989 David Rimmer screened his film *Black Cat White Cat It's a Good
Cat if It Catches the Mouse* for the first time at the International Experimental Film
Congress in Toronto. An experimental documentary about mainland China, it
captures the spirit of the Chinese people's belated emergence into a modern industrial democracy. The news at the time was full of stories about a popular resistance
movement emblematized by the appropriation of the Statue of Liberty as the
Goddess of Democracy. It was the first brief suggestion of the dismantling of a
communist state, and the film enthusiastically confronted the Chinese people as

cultural partners in global communications. Two days later, on 3 June, we heard about Tiananmen Square. Rimmer subsequently added a typescript from Radio Beijing English News Service as a coda to the film. The text gives the details of the massacre, appealing to all radio listeners to join the protest against the barbarous suppression of the people.

The coincidence of this screening and the tragedy in Beijing is significant to an appreciation of David Rimmer's filmmaking. At the congress in Toronto the North American experimental film community appeared to be deeply divided over the theory, history, and practice of avant-garde film.[2] Tensions between political correctness and aesthetic formalism dominated the forum. Rimmer's work, however, disproves the polarization of "generations" which emerged in the wake of the congress. As he has been making experimental films since 1967, he is a key figure in the canon, especially as it has been developed in Canada, and yet Rimmer's work is exceptional in the way it has evolved over the last twenty-five years, expanding the parameters of experimental film. *Black Cat White Cat* is a brilliant example of experimental techniques deployed in a socially and culturally engaged film. The uplifting evocation of the spirit of social transformation that dominates the film only makes the historical coda more deeply felt, and it is significant that Tiananmen Square is a space of culture and tourism in *Black Cat White Cat* rather than politics (the Goddess of Democracy never appears). In this film, as in so much of his work, Rimmer's deep understanding of film language produces a highly poetic contribution to a politics of representation.

It is true that the textual coda of *Black Cat White Cat* is far more direct and "engaged" than most of Rimmer's work. It operates as a "supplement," an excess or appendage, not only of this particular film, but of the oeuvre as a whole, pointing to something which tends otherwise to be repressed by the structural formalism of the films. To say that history is repressed in this work is not, however, to say that it is denied or disavowed. It survives as fragments, as fleeting as that moment in modern Chinese history before Tiananmen Square; and it persists as a politics of representation, visibility, and language. A documentary impulse has always informed Rimmer's experimental films, but as the sheer volume of his imagery has expanded since the mid 1980s, this tendency has taken on a renewed urgency in his work.

Because the films of the last ten years still exhibit many of the key tendencies of structural film, Rimmer's work provides something of an index of the expansion and transformation of the avant-garde in postmodern film culture. "Structural film" was P. Adams Sitney's label for the minimalist experimental film of the late 1960s and early 70s, exemplified by Michael Snow's *Wavelength* (1967). It was a mode of film practice which was ostensibly the most sophisticated refinement of the cinematic medium to its essential purities of camera framing and movement, celluloid surface and texture, and projection indices of light and framing. Fixed camera position, flicker effect, loop printing, and rephotography were the key elements of a form of film in which "shape" took priority over "content."[3] For some it was a film form that almost represented consciousness itself.[4] British critics further theorized what they called structural-materialist film as a reflection on the cinematic apparatus, but in privileging the material signifier and its structuration of the spectator, they also eliminated "signifieds" from discussion.[5]

Few films are in fact as minimal as this description suggests, and yet the idea of structural film became the high-modernist cinematic equivalent to Greenbergian minimalism. Paul Arthur notes that "it is increasingly evident that the *unalloyed* investigation of film's material substrate exists as a tiny chapter in the history of the American avant-garde." Nevertheless, he says, as an aesthetic theory it set up "an oscillating field which bracketed connections between materiality and narrative, between the formal and the social."[6] It may be because Rimmer's work insists on these kinds of connections that it has received so little critical attention. Because the most thorough critical treatments of structural film have been in the context of American independent cinema,[7] Canadian filmmakers – except for Snow – have been largely excluded from the canon. But it is also because Rimmer's version of structural film does not evacuate "content" or "signifieds" in the interest of formal experiments that his work has fallen through the cracks of avant-garde theory and criticism. On one hand, there are ways in which his films reverse and challenge both the metaphysical and materialist presuppositions about structural film. On the other, as we shall see, he is able to transform the structural mode into a politics of representation by bringing it to bear on a wide range of images of people, places, objects, and activities.

Rimmer's films have been described as poetic versions of structuralist-materialist avant-garde film praxis, precisely because of the evocative nature of the imagery. Writers on Rimmer's early films would typically make this observation and then proceed to focus on formal technique, virtually ignoring the effects of content and imagery.[8] It is high time that this imagery is placed in the foreground of critical analysis, as this essay intends to do, in order to appreciate the narrative and social codes that are deconstructed in Rimmer's work. The structural film form should emerge from this analysis as a crucial formal means of decentring the "authorization" of images in cinematic representation. The films from *Bricolage* (1984) to *Local Knowledge* (1992) retain the fixed frame, flicker effect, loop printing, and rephotography of structural film. These devices, however, become the means of representing a subjectivity of perception in the contexts of the chosen imagery.

As Rimmer's image bank has expanded to include the wealth of television, video effects have re-invented the formal techniques of structural film. With the increased volume of found footage, the documentary impulse is strengthened as a formal element in itself, to become a form of historical imagination. *As Seen on TV* (1986) and *Local Knowledge* are especially apocalyptic in tenor, in keeping with a tradition of collage filmmaking that would include Bruce Conner, Arthur Lipsett, Craig Baldwin, and Leslie Thornton. Rimmer's work differs in its approximation of historical time by retaining a strong rhythm of repetition within the collage structure. Narrativity becomes less a structural phenomenon than a mode of intensity as the violence to the image is linked to violence in and of the images and the histories from which they are drawn. The retention of structural film techniques within a complex and often dangerous image-world becomes a representation of a subjectivity which is increasingly placed in question.

Given the decentring tendencies in Rimmer's filmmaking, it is important to deploy a critical model that does not reproduce holistic mythologies of artistic genius, despite the generic conventions of the gallery monograph. The body of Rimmer's work may be linked by more than his name, but it is a fragmented and historical text. As the films continue to change, Rimmer can only be apprehended as a historical subject in a process of continual transformation. In the following pages, the sequence of twenty "experimental" films of varying length is further fragmented into three critical paradigms of landscape, ethnography, and gender.9 As thematic material and stylistic tendencies, these paradigms are posited as intrusions into a twenty-five-year teleology. As critical tools for situating the work within the changes in cultural politics that have occurred over those twenty-five years, they should provide the means of excavating the "contents" of Rimmer's so-called experiments. Like all critical discourse on the avant-garde, this approach may be accused of killing its object, but since the end of avant-garde film has already been declared,10 this murder is offered as a redemptive form of criticism. If, as Paul Mann argues, the avant-garde thrives on its own immolation as it struggles to renew culture,11 we should welcome this crisis as a historical moment in which filmmakers such as Rimmer might be re-visioned.

> The whole history of art is no more than a massive footnote
> to the history of film.[12]

The 1969 film *Landscape* is the pure form, in the best structural tradition, of a theme that informs a great deal of Rimmer's films. A continuous fixed shot of an ocean inlet, it was intended to be rear-projected onto a Plexiglas screen in a suspended wooden picture frame. Through time-lapse photography, a complete day from sunrise to sundown is condensed into seven and a half minutes. *Landscape* takes the great Canadian picture-postcard and re-naturalizes it, animating the scene with the rapid passage of clouds and shadows across the screen and progressive changes in coloration over the course of the "day." The composition in depth, from foreground grasses to two levels of mountains dipping into the centre of the frame, is enhanced by the play of light on the middle-ground water surface which seems to move toward the viewer, while clouds travel rapidly above the horizon line. A critic in 1970 commented: "The film asks for relaxation, for thought, for dreams, for drifting, for humanity."[13] One does indeed become drawn into the scene, addressed more as a participant than a witness.

Bart Testa has argued that Rimmer's landscape films are exemplary of Gaile McGregor's "Wacousta Syndrome." For McGregor, the representation of landscape in Canadian painting and literature exhibits a "garrison mentality," as opposed to the American mythology of the frontier. A characteristic "anxiety about the horizon" is contained in an emphasis on framing and enclosure; a wilderness perceived as threatening and monstrous is held at bay through pictorial compositions in which "the viewer is protected from imaginative participation."[14] Of *Canadian Pacific* (1974), Testa writes: "The enclosing frame and the obstruction of the view by the boxcars in *Canadian Pacific* doubly articulate a Canadian mentality of perception and representation, namely what McGregor terms a 'boxed experience, a distinction between inside and outside.' "[15]

The two *Canadian Pacific* films – the second (*Canadian Pacific II* [1975]) shot from a window slightly higher than the first, overlooking British Columbia's Burrard Inlet – are composed, like *Landscape*, in depth. Railway cars in the foreground, ships in the middle ground, and snow-covered mountains in the distance create a landscape that is thoroughly industrialized, as the title, which appears on several boxcars, suggests. Both films include weather stripping around the window frame, as a frame-within-the-frame, and both films end with the camera capturing its own reflection on the darkened window of nightfall. Losing the light, losing the image, the cinematic apparatus is redundant, having nothing but itself to film. The strict separation of inside and outside in the two *Canadian Pacific* films may indeed suggest a garrison mentality, and yet both formal composition and the narrativization of daylight also refer to the structure of the gaze within the landscape.

Landscape in *Canadian Pacific I* and *II*, as in *Landscape*, completes the look, and is an extension of a gaze which in turn domesticates the scene of nature. Nature does not thereby become a "garden" (with its connotations of being tamed and controlled), but becomes a patterned, textured environmental space that changes according to the viewpoint from which it is framed. Far from being "monstrous," it becomes a home for the eye, a restful and welcoming sight that reaches forward to the vanishing points of the perspective, completing a structure of representation that includes and is predicated on the viewing subject-position. In splitting the vantage point over two films in *Canadian Pacific I* and *II*, and in contextualizing both scene and seer as industrialized and technologized, the construction of subjectivity is materialist rather than idealist.[16] Neither the "eye" of the camera nor the "nature" of landscape becomes a symbolic property, but both are bound into an apparatus of perception.

Despite the framing and inhabited foreground, two characteristics of McGregor's Wacousta Syndrome, it is difficult to see any evidence of a garrison mentality in Rimmer's landscape films. Testa's reading of the films not only misses the aesthetic point of Rimmer's treatment of landscape, but it also belittles the regional specificity of his West Coast reference points. In the interests of a "Canadian identity," McGregor's highly reductive and ahistorical formalism mimics the worst features of the American mythology it aims to counter. It ignores the vital differences within Canadian culture, and it belittles the vast differences within the Canadian landscape, which are significant to the various Canadian regions.

A more appropriate context for the representation of landscape in Rimmer's films might be found in the local art history of Vancouver. Similar treatments of landscape can be found in the work of some of Rimmer's contemporaries in the visual arts, such as Tom Burrows's *Untitled* (1971)[17] and Dean Ellis's *Grounds* (1974).[18] One can also include in a history of landscape painting in Vancouver the Group of Seven painters F.H. Varley and Lawren Harris, as well as Emily Carr and

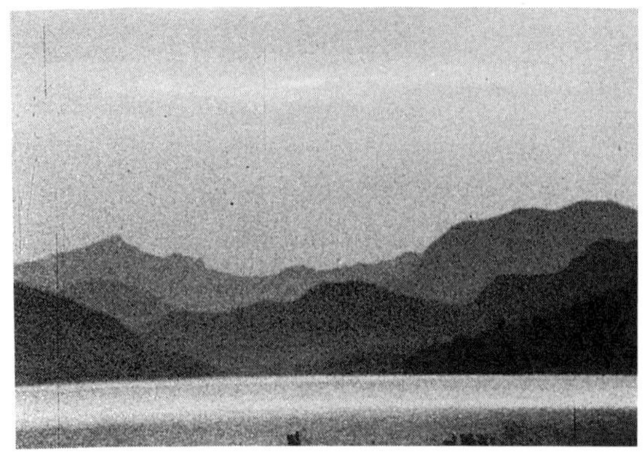

Landscape 1969

The Dance 1970

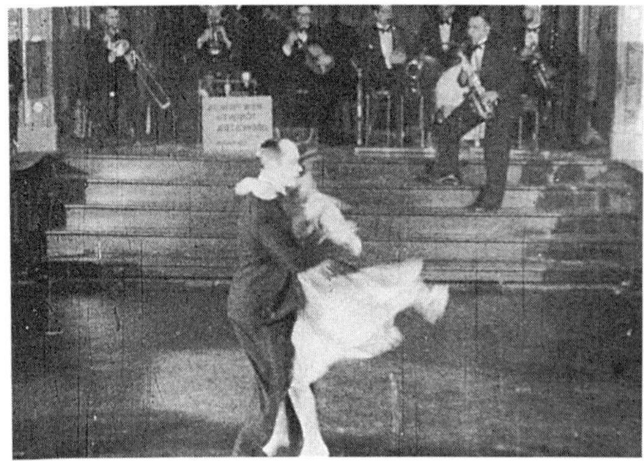

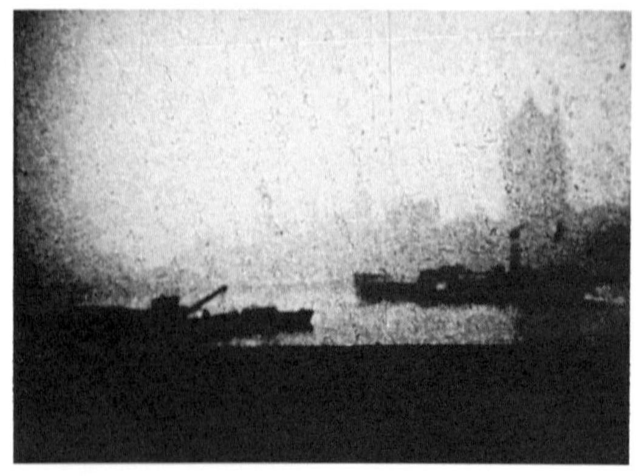

Surfacing on the Thames 1970

Variations on a Cellophane Wrapper 1970

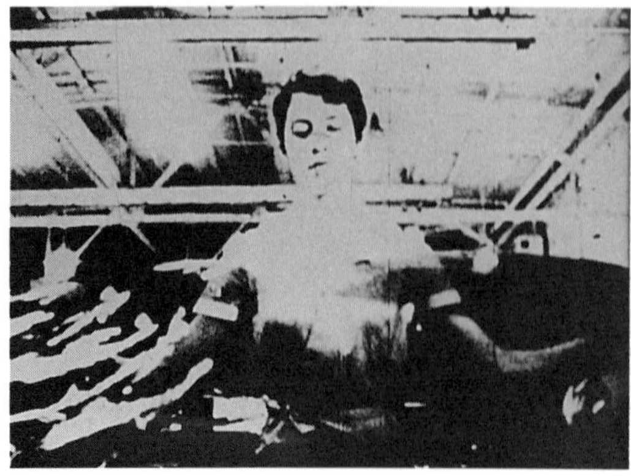

the abstract expressionist landscapes of Jack Shadbolt, Takao Tanabe, and Gordon Smith. Living in a remote outpost of a colonial culture, British Columbian artists who originated "somewhere else" have looked to their dramatic landscape for a sense of place and identity.[19]

One can no doubt find traces of McGregor's "themes" in Carr's dense forests and Varley's *Open Window* (1933), but what McGregor reads in the Manichaean terms of hostile nature/safe enclosure can often also be read as a domestication of the wilderness – domestication, not as a "taming" but as a being-at-home-within, an inhabitation. Scott Watson says of the Vancouver painting of the 1950s:

> It is ironic that the heroic, individualistic myth informing the New Yorkers often resorted to a nineteenth century image of man in the frontier while on the actual frontier, a place like Vancouver, the image is in the urban present tense.... [T]he painting of this period, although it has been characterized as landscape – by Shadbolt, Reid and others – is best understood as part of the desire to "become cosmopolitan."... [T]he "landscape" element of the Vancouver fifties painters was a compositional device, used to make images that refer to interior emotions as much as, if not more than, exterior places.[20]

Rimmer's structural film technique, refined in New York from 1970 to 1974, is brought home to bear on the local scene in a very literal way. Like the Group of Seven's modernism and the abstract expressionism of the 1950s in British Columbia, it has the effect of familiarizing a landscape which is distinctively West Coast and making a place within it, transforming a "vista" into an environment.

The perspectival compositions of the *Canadian Pacific* films and *Landscape* are complicated somewhat in *Narrows Inlet* (1980), a film in which the camera pans back and forth, completing at least one 360-degree movement around an unidentified centre. Unlike Michael Snow's *La région centrale* (1971), these camera movements are random and swinging, as if the camera were mounted on a boat. Wooden pilings in the middle ground are evidence again of an inhabited natural environment, and the first half of the film is so drenched with mist and fog that the shore and rising mountains of the background are entirely hidden. When the lushly coloured pine forests emerge from the blue-grey fog, a Group of Seven landscape appears to emerge from a more abstract expressionist surface composition of line and texture. The horizontal pans inscribe a centralized but unstable point of vision, constructing a shifting, apparently "floating" subjectivity within this

painterly landscape. All three films thus represent landscape as a phenomenological production of an invisible but determining seeing camera/subject/viewer.
Landscape depends on point of view, and at the same time extends and embodies
that point of view as part of its nature.

Landscape in Rimmer's films is also much more than framing and horizon
lines. It is a dynamic space of movement and light, often captured by time-lapse
cinematography. The patterns and rhythms of cloud movement and the play of
light and shadow over water surfaces are further examples of the domestication of
the natural environment. A certain familiarity with landscape is evoked by the
cycles of weather patterns and daylight that structure many of the films. In the later
films *Along the Road to Altamira* (1986), *Black Cat White Cat*, and *Local Knowledge*,
landscape tends to be lit with sunsets and sunrises, and functions as a powerful
index of change, transformation, and travel. In *Black Cat White Cat*, the Chinese
landscape is repeatedly shot from a moving train, often as the sun sinks behind a
silhouetted forest. This fiery imagery is fundamental to the film's sense of social
and historical movement. Towards the end, a huge industrial landscape is similarly
silhouetted by a horizontal camera movement at sunset.

The title graphics in all three films crawl across the screen horizontally,
announcing the filmic practice as a trajectory taking place in the time of travel and
the space of landscape. In *Altamira*, the titles travel across the darkened bottom of
an image of the sun rising over a desert horizon, to a light Spanish guitar soundtrack. Using various structural filmic techniques, this film represents the tourist
experience as a fragmentary and decentred quest for an impossible knowledge of
time and space. A rapid montage of postcards of Mont Saint-Michel collapses a
multitude of perspectives into a single image. In seeking an alternative to this
commodification of landscape, the filmic trajectory is towards the cave paintings
of Altamira. The barely discernible drawings are a surface form of representation,
and the rephotographed Super-8 film of the cave tends to conflate the screen surface with the cave wall. The tourist's quest for authentic spectacle ends, finally,
with a very literal inscription on the inverted landscape of the prehistoric rock face.
Landscape usually implies depth of field, which is called into question by a natural
sight/site that lacks perspective.

Local Knowledge is organized around the most complex representation of landscape, extending the surface/depth dialectic, as well as the patterns and metaphors
of weather and sunlight, into an epic form. The title refers to the familiarity with
landscape necessary to uncharted navigation in coastal waters. An image of a West

Coast inlet surrounded by mountains dipping into the middle distance recurs throughout this densely textured film. In fact, this is the same scene as the one in *Landscape*, Skookumchuck Rapids, leading out of Storm Bay to the ocean beyond. Shot from the water, above the prow of a motorboat speeding into the centre where the horizon seems to part and reveal an opening, the scene is one of security and home, especially when it recurs after sequences of mysterious and slightly threatening imagery. Again, it is the composition in depth, from a fixed vantage point which appears to be entering into and being received by the landscape, that breaks down mythic dualities of insides and outsides, nature and technology.

This coastal landscape is also shot from other, less stable, less secure perspectives, radically transformed by fog, by clouds swirling in time-lapse movements, and by sunsets. The sun keeps going down in *Local Knowledge*, making the broad-daylight shots from the boat all the more comforting. An ominous soundtrack of Asian and electronic instrumentation increases the sense of foreboding as the landscape is lost again and again to darkness. Another key image of the film is a stand of trees behind which sunsets are reflected in rapid overhead cloud movements. This image has been digitalized in video and, as a frame-within-the-frame, revolves on a central axis at the beginning and end of the film. As it does to so much of the imagery, video flattens the scene onto a two-dimensional surface, highlighted in this case by special effects.

Breaking down images in video and rephotographing them in film makes them literally "weathered." The grain of the image, which in Rimmer's films since *Canadian Pacific* has been somewhat analogous to the effect of weather on landscape (fog, rain, and mist), becomes a sign of transformation. The meeting of videography and landscape in *Local Knowledge* evokes not just formal transformation or mediation, but social and historical change of revolutionary and apocalyptic dimensions. In one shot, distinctively marked by video tracking signals, trees can be seen bending in violent winds (the footage is u.s. Army documentation of an atomic blast). Combined with further ambiguous and threatening representations of violence and technological weather – a weather station surrounded by barbed wire, and a military weather report – the weather in this film becomes an iconography of danger and inevitability. It does so in part because of the codes of tv news embedded in its videographed representation.

In stark contrast to the landscape shots of *Local Knowledge*, a repeated image of fish fills the frame with a mass of writhing bodies. The flatness of the image is enhanced by superimposed geometric graphics, dialectically related to the depth of the mass. Intercut with shots of water surfaces, the fish suggest both the "repressed" content of the ocean and the erotics of the unconscious. Disorienting and vaguely disturbing, the image points to the industrial exploitation of the coastal waters and also to another depth besides that of depth-of-field. As another videographed image, it pushes the structural film's preoccupation with screen surface to a certain paradoxical extreme, radically obliterating horizon(tal) space.

Blue Movie (1970), a study of ocean waves and clouds, is completely without framing devices, perspectival markers, or anything besides water and sky – not even a horizon. It is a study of the kind of image that Snow's long zoom dissolves into at the end of *Wavelength*, an image of no dimensions, no perspective, no subjectivity. Camera angles and solarization flatten the water surface as the waves become patterns of movement, colour, and light. While this level of abstraction returns for brief moments in later films, it tends to be contextualized in order to refer back to the subject of vision. *Local Knowledge* contains a quick upside-down shot of water rushing under (or over, as the case may be) a boat-mounted camera with the sky on the bottom of the frame. The disorientation it produces is echoed in another shot from the stern of a boat travelling away from the shore; the reverse-action photography depicts a certain stasis, a rapid movement that goes nowhere. Landscape, along with its various inversions, becomes a vital substance of vision for an iconography of emplacement, familiarity, and transformation.

Surfacing on the Thames (1970) is Rimmer's most exacting experiment with movement in landscape, which in this case is the remote and foreign London skyline. The passage of a boat across the fixed frame, broken down into constitutive frames that are then dissolved into each other, is a retarded and almost mystical motion. Surface and depth take on historical significance as we look through the scratches and flaws of the rephotographed film to the found footage below. Critics have pointed out the resemblance of the slightly unfocused scene to Turner's painting, and to the pointillists, and it is indeed an ironically romantic effect which is created through an analysis of the materiality of the film medium.[21] Rimmer's films often aspire to the condition of painting by way of imagery composed around a horizon, but even in *Surfacing*, that horizon refers to a subject of vision: the zoom out of the centre of the image at the beginning of the film, and in again at the end, penetrate the illusion of depth to reveal its dependency on structures of perception and composition. The use of dissolves in *Surfacing* is a device which few of Rimmer's contemporary structural filmmakers used, and one which he favours in many of the later films, especially *Local*

Knowledge. Dissolving images into each other is a means of merging film and landscape in this early prototype of cinematic "weathering."

Nature and technology tend to be thoroughly combined in Rimmer's films. Their dualism is transcended in the deconstruction of perspectival vision implicit in his structural film form, and the phenomenology of camera-vision is turned back on itself. In her discussion of *Wavelength*, Annette Michelson refers to the "'horizon' characteristic of every subjective process and fundamental as a trait of intentionality" to explain the constitution of the viewer in time.[22] When "horizon" is literalized in landscape, spatial determinants take priority over temporal ones and the viewer is located spatially within the perspective and the film. In the very limited freedom of. the fixed camera position, the phenomenological "transcendental subject" is referred to, but not mobilized. The view of nature unsettles the instrumentalized gaze, rendering it dependent on the scene itself, which, through darkness and weather, also limits the field of vision. Landscape is a vehicle of and for movement, the movement of history and industry, and it is a receptacle for the eye, a home for vision, until it is transferred to video. With the loss of depth, the technologized landscape takes on a threatening demeanour, a vaguely discomforting two-dimensionality. Even in *Local Knowledge*, though, this apocalyptic postmodernism is counterbalanced by recurring images of the security of a West Coast inlet.

Ethnography: The Populated Frame

Otherness becomes empowering critical difference when it is not given, but re-created.[23]

None of Rimmer's films can be described as "ethnographic films," and yet people figure as importantly as landscape in his oeuvre. Neither characters nor documentary subjects, people's images are visually explored and examined with an intensity and epistemological distance equal to that of the ethnographer. My use of the term ethnography should, however, be distinguished from the authoritative disciplinary context in which it originated as a branch of anthropology. Ethnography refers here to what James Clifford describes as "diverse ways of thinking and writing about culture from a standpoint of participant observation."[24] Rimmer's interest in people and culture is in this sense symptomatic of what Clifford describes as "a pervasive postcolonial crisis of ethnographic authority":

> A modern "ethnography" of conjuncture, constantly moving *between* cultures, does not, like its Western alter-ego "anthropology," aspire to survey the full range of human diversity or development. It is perpetually displaced, both regionally focused and broadly comparative, a form both of dwelling and travel in a world where the two experiences are less and less distinct.[25]

Three separate tendencies in Rimmer's films impinge on ethnography: found film footage of people in historically distant cultures, travel footage, and TV imagery (including film transferred to video). In each case, the cultural "other" is silenced, observed, and often radically objectified through the manipulation of the image. Reserving analysis of the role of gender in this process for the last section of this essay, the structures of voyeurism can here be analyzed as they pertain to historical and ethnographic imagery. I do not want to imply that Rimmer's films are voyeuristic, but rather that they deconstruct the epistemological politics of voyeurism implicit in structural film's foregrounding of the apparatus.[26] Andy Warhol's structural films of the 1960s are the most important precursors of such a practice, but whereas Warhol counters voyeurism with the exhibitionism of the film and fashion industries, Rimmer allegorizes voyeurism as historiography and tourism.

The Dance (1970), *Seashore* (1971), and *Watching for the Queen* (1973) are all short films, each of which is built upon a single piece of found footage of people performing some kind of activity. The brief gesture or movement is repeated in loops that function somewhat differently in each of the three films. Although the source of the image is unknown in *Seashore*, the bourgeois settings and costume, the composition in depth, and the quotidian action are highly evocative of the Lumières' style and era.[27] To describe it as ethnographic is to draw a tacit parallel between the myths of primitivism which inform both avant-garde film and traditional ethnography. Structural filmmakers' preoccupation with early cinema was part and parcel of the introspective "purification" of the medium. The stripping away of institutional and narrative codes led numerous filmmakers back to cinema's origins where pictorial composition, montage (or the lack thereof), and

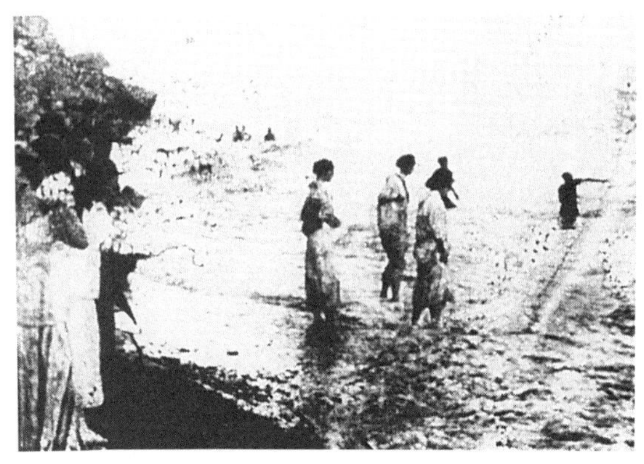

Seashore 1971

Fracture 1973

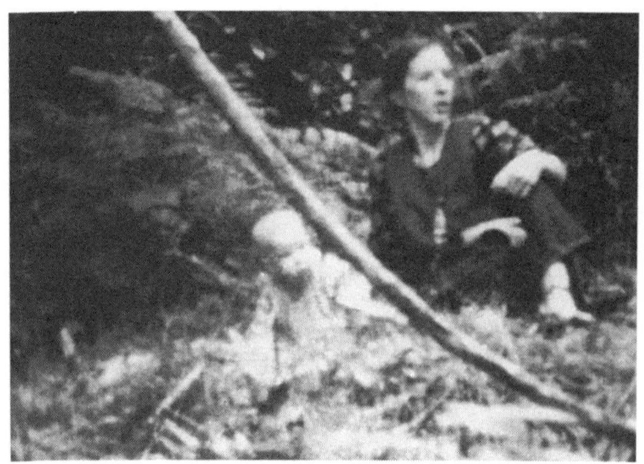

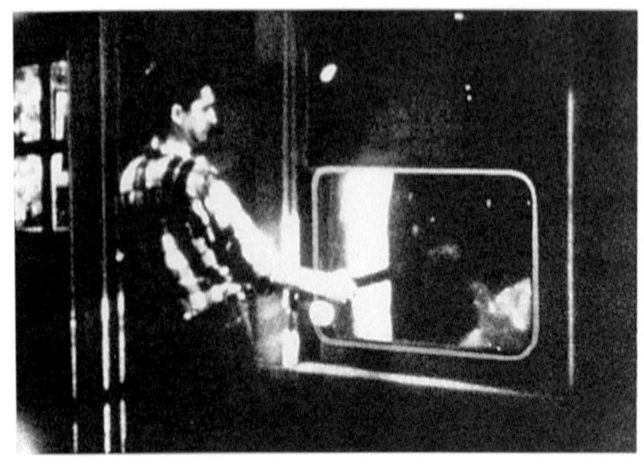

Bricolage 1984

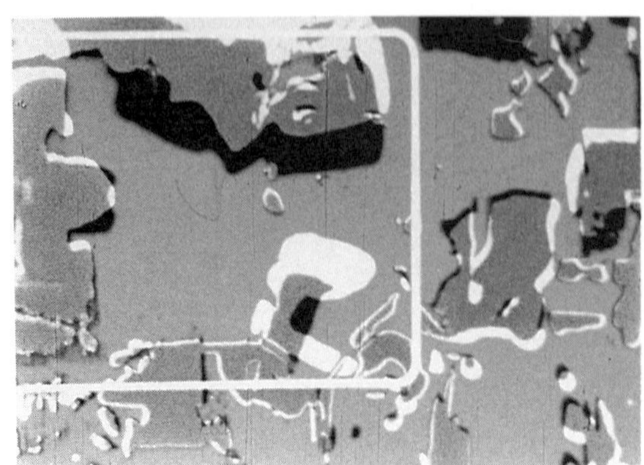

address might be found in their raw state, uncontaminated by "bourgeois" narrative codes. Bart Testa describes avant-garde appropriations of early cinema as "pedagogical interventions, as works that allow us to see cinema again, in places and at levels where we had ceased to see it."[28]

The fragment of film upon which Rimmer works in *Seashore* has been related by Testa to "the many picturesque views of the sea, boats and the shore in the first years of film production ... [whose] composition in large measure defined the visual code of the extreme long shot."[29] The fragment in *Seashore* consists of four groups of figures: three women in the centre tentatively wade into the sea, a couple of bathers screen-right play in the waves, a group of men and women stand fully dressed on the shore screen-left, and a group of bathers waist-deep in the middle distance stand off a rocky outcrop completing the curve of the beach. It is a complex image with a number of rhythms, including the movement of the water. When the loop is shortened, the smaller movements and gestures appear automatic and mechanical; when the fragment is flipped and superimposed on the original screen direction, the image becomes symmetrically framed. A total fragmentation of the image occurs with the imitation of projection flaws: white leader, frame lines, and flicker.

All of these formal devices, added to the pattern of surface flaws on the film emphasized by freeze-frames, distract the viewer from the original image. Testa concludes his analysis by pointing out that "Rimmer has brought a distinction between recorded event, however literally or lyrically rendered, and the limited compositional stability of the perspective system in cinema."[30] With the destabilization of the composition, the recorded event becomes more indistinct and more distant, a distance which is historical before it is ethnographic. Rimmer's rephotography of found footage is allegorical in the sense that its signified content lies elsewhere, in another movie in another time.[31] That "other time" may be a mythic time in film history, but simultaneously, the historical referent has the specificity of the singular moment captured by a seaside photographer.

The affinities between history and ethnography are crucial to the mythology of primitivism. Clifford explains: "The salvage paradigm, reflecting a desire to rescue 'authenticity' out of destructive historical change, is alive and well. It is found not only in ethnographic writing but also in the connoisseurships and collections of the art world and in a range of familiar nostalgias."[32] The designation of early cinema as primitive cinema by Noël Burch is a good example of this practice, which more recent historians have been quick to point out.[33] Pre-Griffith cinema is "primitive" because, like "primitive" cultures, it preserves something "essential" in its naïveté. Burch's formalist historiography imposes a modernist antibourgeois aesthetic onto a body of work that was produced in very different historical circumstances. The historiography of early cinema has tended, by and large, to repress, or at least subordinate, questions of imagery and codes of signification to questions of form.

At first glance, structural film practice might appear to do the same, and yet it is more difficult to ignore the people who populated early cinema when they cross your field of vision, and cross it again and again and again. The almost accidental emergence of a trace of history – real people doing real things – is the obverse of the salvage paradigm which tends to endow the historically and culturally specific with meanings well beyond the documented experience (meanings of primitivism, of anthropological humanism, of pastoral romanticism, etc.). Instead of "bringing culture into writing," which for Clifford is the enactment of the structure of "salvage,"[34] *Seashore* discovers culture already written and investigates the structure of this representation. It reproduces the allegorical structure of ethnography in such a way that writing – the language of representation – is shown to destroy and violate the referent.

The brevity and anonymity of the fragment of history that is glimpsed in *Seashore* might seem to compromise its epistemological value. And yet its connotative meaning is rich precisely because it is "foreign" and difficult to decode. What are the relationships between the different groups of people? Is the group on the beach crowded into the frame because they are posing? Are the bathers in the water male or female, young or old? Is this a typical leisure activity of this period, whatever period it is? In this country, whatever country it is? Precisely because these questions have no answers, a level of inquisition is denied and subordinated to a more respectful attitude of passive observation. The privilege of looking into history is itself finally taken away in the reduction of the image to light, line, and form.

Watching for the Queen may have an opposite trajectory to that of *Seashore*, restoring a "whole" film fragment from its composite frames, but it is no less a reversal of the salvage paradigm. In this case the image is of a crowd looking into the camera, as if the filmmaker and we who necessarily adopt the camera's gaze, were the queen. The two-second shot of the crowd is looped at progressively faster speeds, from one minute for the first frame, slowly working up to the "normal" speed of twenty-four frames per second, so that the narrative of *Watching* is the reconstruction of the original shot. The film creates a sort of mirror effect as we watch for the crowd to do their watching, and it provokes a certain pleasure when this is accomplished, when the crowd finally moves "like a crowd" united, like us, in their mutual fascination. Because of the slight tilt of the camera, one has to scan the image to relocate figures from one frame to the next. A man near the centre of the image wearing a military-style cap raises his head in one of the largest gestures of the group to meet our gaze, but as he does, his movement is lost in the general jostling of the crowd. If the freezing of individual frames allows us to discern individuals within the mass of faces that fills the screen, the restoration of movement denies the autonomy of their gestures and redefines the group as one that moves together in a single swaying gesture.

As ethnography, this film is as ambiguous as *Seashore,* and one tends to place a great deal of semantic weight on the title. Whether these people are really watching for the queen or not, the title refers us to the practice of spectatorship and the panopticonic form of an apparatus which retains control even when authority is the ostensible object of scrutiny.[35] Placing the crowd under microscopic analysis in *Watching* represents a relation of empowerment and subordination that the title obliquely associates with a colonial relationship. The monarchy may be the ostensible spectacle, but its image is withheld, and the representation of power is extended into a technology of power. The crowd's subservience to the monarchic gaze is analyzed as a mechanism of representation in which cinema becomes an allegory for the irreversible structure of voyeurism. It isolates the subject-effect of ethnography as an abstraction of individuality and an imbalance of power which can, nevertheless, be apprehended as a technology. The triumphant moment of closure is one in which the viewer realizes that his or her constitution as a subject of vision is dependent on the loss of subjectivities on the part of the people in the image; we necessarily adopt the point of view of "the queen," protected by invisibility.

The Dance may be less ethnographic than the other two films because the original film fragment is of a performance rather than the quotidian activities of *Seashore* and *Watching.* The stage setting is itself exaggerated by opening and closing shots of a theatre audience applauding, shot from the perspective of a stage across which a curtain opens and closes. But the dance itself, a couple jiving in front of a jazz band, is more likely set in a 1940s nightclub than a "legitimate" theatre. The disjunction between audience and show is in keeping with the central trick of the film: the dancers repeat a six-second movement back and forth across the stage while the soundtrack is a continuous piece of music. The dissynchrony is humorous, and the irony is at the expense of the poor musicians and dancers who are caught in an endless series of identical gestures until they are finally released from the repetition with the closing chords of the piece. Like so much comedy, there is a certain cruelty involved, this time with respect to the integrity of the original performance and performers.

While *The Dance* exhibits a certain self-conscious flair for presentation, adopting the performative codes of the dance for its own "brilliant" execution of technique, the ironic tone provides another counter-gesture to the salvage paradigm. The specificity of the historical and cultural setting of the dance resists appropriation: it is ironically endowed with an anonymity that such footage typically lacks. As in *Seashore* and *Watching*, repetition functions as a vehicle of amplification for a fragment of film that is only "meaningful" insofar as it is different from our own cultural and historical experience. Even the mirror-effect of *Watching* is destabilized by the black-and-white footage which, in invoking an archival past, differentiates the people as cultural others. In each case, the formal experiments are performed within an ethnographic structure of perception and power, a structure discovered to be a technology and an apparatus through its deconstruction.

In each of these films, and also in the many other examples of found footage throughout Rimmer's work, the anonymity of the people filmed is made mysterious. The images tend to evoke a sense which Roland Barthes has described in *Camera Lucida*: "Since every photograph is contingent (and thereby outside of meaning), Photography cannot signify (aim at a generality) except by assuming a mask."[36] Photographic contingency "immediately yields up those 'details' which constitute the very raw material of ethnological knowledge."[37] And yet Rimmer never allows us the time for contemplation necessary to the pleasure of the photographic text. The movement, repetitions, and fragmentation of the image provoke a desire for a look which is always denied by the filmic appropriation of the photographed scene.

The films flirt with photography and its freeze-frame cinematic version (especially *Watching*), and in this flirtation allude to the that-has-been of the photographic referent.[38] Because they allude to it, though, without touching it, without stopping to gaze wistfully into the past (with the possible exception of *Surfacing*), an allegorical structure is maintained. The "primitive" form of the *Seashore* fragment belongs to a history apprehended as distant, but also different. Photography may have "something to do with resurrection,"[39] but no such mythology informs Rimmer's historical ethnography. Faces are summoned up from the archive for our viewing pleasure, but their masks remain secure and they remain dead. If they weren't dead already, as in the case of the vibrant dancers in *The Dance*, they are killed by the violence of the cutting. Refusing the "sting" of the *punctum*, that detail which for Barthes reaches out of the photograph and grabs the viewer in his or her present tense, is also a denial of the mythology of salvage: that "we" are like "them."[40]

A very different construction of otherness is inscribed in *Real Italian Pizza*, shot in New York from September 1970 to May 1971. This is not only Rimmer's most overtly ethnographic film, but because of the setting, it also serves as a foil or counterpole to Snow's *Wavelength*. Outside the loft window he finds the life of the street which Snow so radically excludes. Turning the camera onto the patrons of an Italian pizza and sandwich shop, their rhythms of coming and going and just hanging out on the sidewalk, Rimmer assumes the position of the spy. From his elevated angle, across the street, the New Yorkers, many of them African-American, look like ants or bees revolving around a buzzing hive. Another kind of "queen," the pizza-makers/shop-owners remain invisible. They come out once to shovel snow off the sidewalk, but for the most part, their invisibility and centrality on the other side of the scenario mirrors and complements that of the camera.[41]

Each of the three overlapping camera positions in the film has the effect of framing the scene like a stage onto which people exit and enter. Collapsing nine months into thirteen minutes, Rimmer's editing exaggerates the rhythms and patterns of the routines of daily life, lingering on those who loiter outside the shop during the summer months, pixilating rapid activity, and when the police drag someone out of the shop, dramatically cutting into the scene to see the apprehended man stuffed into a patrol car. The brief shot is the proverbial exception which proves the rule of the otherwise statically framed film. In comparison to many of Rimmer's films, the "real" documentary image is more or less sustained in its integrity. Although it is step-printed and looped in order to exaggerate the senses of rapid activity and routine, it also comes close to the candid *verité* technique of observation. Moreover, when that observational technique is combined with the structural adherence to the fixed frame, the investigative thrust of *cinéma verité* ethnography (as in the work of Jean Rouch or Pierre Perrault) is exposed in its derailment.

Despite the intervention into the image by way of montage and the addition of a jazz soundtrack, Rimmer's camera is extremely passive. Again, this should be contrasted to Snow's zoom inside the loft. The voyeurism of the film's premise is met by the exhibitionism of some of the shop's patrons who, on a couple of occasions, dance on the sidewalk. Although their steps are almost synched to the film's soundtrack, the silencing of their own transistor music retains the distanciation of the spectacle. The scene of the sidewalk is a public space which is specific to New York, and is therefore an ethnographic "sight." Likewise, the people on the street may be "villagers" (inhabitants of a neighbourhood), but they are also there "to be seen." The scene may be outside the filmmaker's window, but it is also – like *Canadian Pacific* – an extension of that New York window.[42]

Real Italian Pizza is an unusual example of ethnographic poetics in experimental film, idiosyncratically suspended as it is between two very different film practices – structural film and *cinéma verité*. The soundtrack of jazz music and traffic sounds helps to accentuate a rhythm of life which is both daily and seasonal. As in any ethnographic text, the film imposes a form and a structure on cultural others in the very process of transposing them into representation. And yet the fixed camera of structural film has the effect of "framing" that process, and quite literally inscribing its limits. Twenty years later, the afros, the bell-bottoms, and the dance-steps are documents of a historically specific culture that occupied a certain public space. Racial difference is embraced within ethnographic difference, which is in turn represented as a spatial difference inscribed within a technology of perception. The form of the film makes the scene into a spectacular other, just as the twenty intervening years make us now into historical voyeurs, looking but not touching, outside the scene looking in, inside the window looking out.

When Rimmer goes to China in *Black Cat White Cat*, a similar fixed-frame *verité* shooting style, combined with atmospheric, ethnographic music, helps to negotiate the representation of more radical cultural difference. The imagery at the beginning of the film might be described as conventionally ethnographic, especially the faces isolated in crowds and the trancelike tai chi witnessed very voyeuristically through trees. The stylized underlit setting of the tai chi, accompanied by Chinese music, is an exotic – even Orientalist – treatment which by the end of the film is reversed. When the Chinese tourists in Tiananmen square crowd around the camera, presumably staring at Rimmer, he is representing himself and his perspective as touristic rather than ethnographic. In doing so, he shares something with his ostensible subjects, as he repeatedly finds the Chinese people to be tourists also: at the Great Wall, at the Forbidden City, at a park or cemetery. None of these places are named as historic sites, but are represented as anonymous "sights" enjoyed by Chinese and foreigners alike.

No foreigners actually appear in the film, but the English language is omnipresent, especially in the language lessons heard on the soundtrack. Among

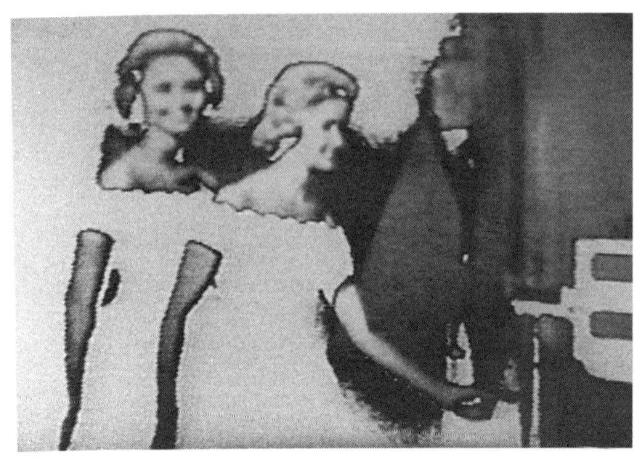

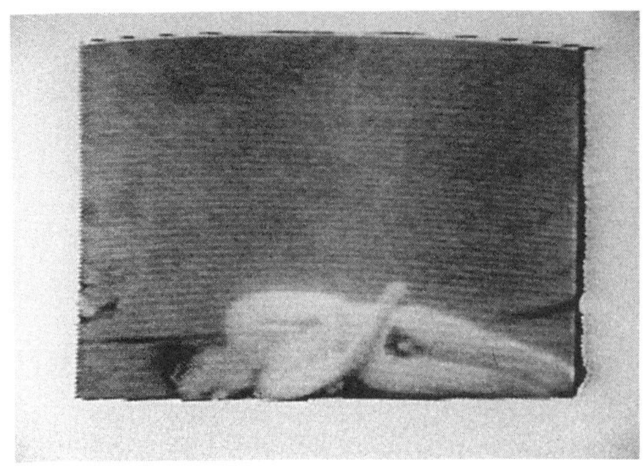

As Seen on TV 1986

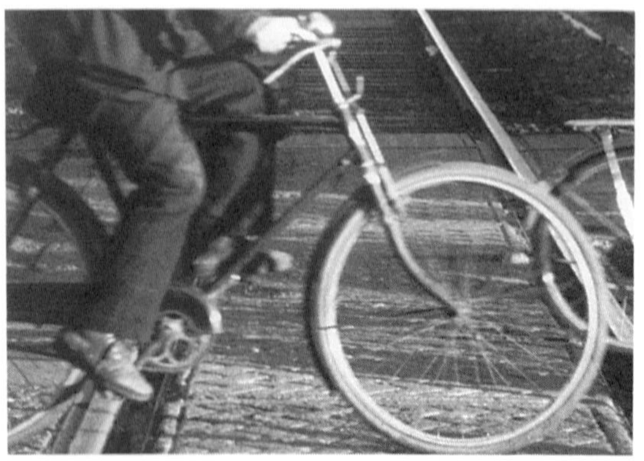

Black Cat White Cat It's a Good Cat if It Catches the Mouse 1989

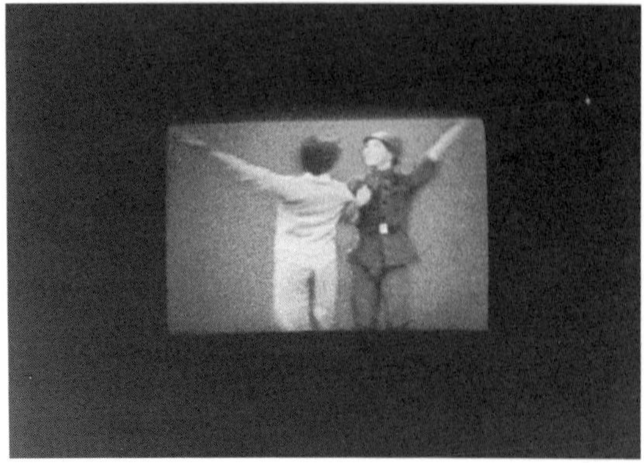

the fragments of phrases and narratives articulated in perfect, if halting, English is a woman describing a medical examination. An odd and disturbing parallel between technology, language, and a violation of the body is suggested. While she speaks, we see a billboard advertising "White Cat low-foaming detergent" in English with Chinese characters. Trinh T. Minh-ha is critical of the "incorporation (if not emphasis) of recognizable signs of Westernization" in ethnographic film, for exoticism can only be consumed when it is salvaged, that is reappropriated and translated into the Master's language of authenticity. A difference that *defies while not defying* is not exotic, it is not even recognized as difference, it is simply no language to the dominant's ear.[43]

The prevalence of English in *Black Cat White Cat* is neither authentic nor authoritative, but serves as a sign of neocolonialism which is at the same time a sign of capitalism and technological modernism. It draws the tourist's eye and ear to signs by which the filmmaker locates himself (and by fiat, his non-Chinese viewer) as a foreigner to the culture. It is the English which is being consumed as exotic within a quotidian Chinese context. Between the aesthetics of exoticism and the technology of salvage lies an ethnographic poetics of passivity in which a strong subjective presence is inscribed. The camera placed on a railway crossing is stationary in a steady stream of bicycle traffic, but the shifts in depth of field effected by the proximity of the passing vehicles and cyclists refer back to the perspectival system anchored to the observer.

The trajectory of *Black Cat White Cat* from the opening image of an inked finger carefully writing the film's title in Chinese characters, to a montage of television imagery, is, as I have already suggested, one of social transformation. The recurring punctuating shots of sunsets glimpsed from a moving train inscribe a sense of historicity and movement, but it is above all in the terms of language that the "other culture" is seen to be in the throes of rapid change. Glimpses of Shanghai TV reveal a culture rich in performance codes and complex intertextuality, a culture of spoken, written, and body language. One is immersed in its signifiers, and it flows over one like a river over a floating stick. Referentiality is in constant flux as every shot refers back to the observer failing to understand the language heard or the activity observed. The social movement is not towards Westernization or capitalism, but into some new and different modern culture with different traditions.

It should be clear by now that Rimmer's work is ethnographic in ways that stretch the term well beyond its usual meaning. While there is a huge difference between the use of found footage in *Seashore* and the cultural encounter of *Black Cat White Cat*, thinking of both tendencies as ethnographic specifies the documentary thrust of Rimmer's films. The gaze at other people is often direct, and as we shall see in the next section, is often returned. Breaking down distinctions between voyeurism and exhibitionism is key to tempering ethnographic ethics and power relations. Photographing television imagery in *As Seen on TV* and *Local Knowledge* is yet another means of looking directly at randomly selected, decontextualized people performing unusual activities. Video in Rimmer's films is the sign of institutionalized mediation, of an authorized glimpse into other worlds, cultures, and lives, of which he takes full advantage. In *Local Knowledge* and *Divine Mannequin* (1989), he even transfers his own footage of objects and landscape onto video and then back into film, producing a sign of mediation within the image itself.

One of the final images of *Local Knowledge* is an outtake of *Black Cat White Cat* – a woman performing tai chi, or possibly dancing, but she is not a dancer and is not on a stage. She does not exhibit herself the way the women do on TV. Decelerated to quarter-speed and videographed, the shot lingers on screen longer than any other in the film. Ethnographic filmmakers have long been attracted to the trance or possession dance as particularly cinematic, perhaps because of the way it blurs the distinction between exhibitionist performance and investigative observation, an objectification of a remote subjectivity. It bears these connotations here, as an oasis of calm meditation within a montage of violent and dramatic imagery. Although *Local Knowledge* is not a travel film, it travels widely through a kaleidoscope of imagery in order to return again and again to a familiar landscape. The tension between coming and going, encapsulated in the temporally reversed shot of landscape from the back of a boat, may not be so different from the tension of staring at someone so "at home" with themselves that they can display their body so gracefully in a public park. In one case you are not really going anywhere, and in the other, you are not really seeing anything. Perhaps this is the melancholia of the film.

The title, *Local Knowledge,* is also Clifford Geertz's, but it means something quite different for the anthropologist and the filmmaker. For Geertz, local knowledge is a technique of explaining social phenomena by "placing them in local frames of awareness"[44] as opposed to imposing epistemological or interpretive schemas upon them. For Rimmer, these frames of awareness are never available. Everything is out of place except one's own home, which is itself only a frame of awareness. The flaw in Geertz's theory is of course his failure to account for his knowledge of other local knowledges and the mediation implicit in his acquisition of that "knowledge."[45] Rimmer's ethnography never ventures into epistemological terrain, but by remaining outside looking in, many of his films work closely with ethnographic strategies in a poetics of "self-fashioning," in which one comes to know oneself through the encounter with others.

"Ethnographic subjectivity," argues James Clifford, "is composed of participant observation in a world of 'cultural artifacts' linked ... to a new conception of language – or better, languages – seen as discrete systems of signs."[46] Rimmer's encounter with others always refers back to himself through the cinematic apparatus and its inscription of subjectivity. At the same time, this apparatus registers the world as forms of language, in which all identities are fictions and every image alludes to unknown identities. The filmmaker's encounter with others, at once insistent and passive, is also a construction of self within a heterogeneous cultural landscape.

Gender: The Discontented Image

THE BIRTH OF A DAUGHTER IS LIKE RECEIVING A BLOSSOM.

– Beijing wall poster, quoted in *Black Cat White Cat*

In *Variations on a Cellophane Wrapper* (1970) a woman in a factory lifts a huge sheet of transparent material which flutters across her body, catching the light. The brief shot, the only image in the film, is cut and repeated just at the moment she lifts her eyes from the table. In the subsequent repetitions, the image is solarized and abstracted in a virtuoso display of technical effects that eventually break it down into an abstract display of line, colour, and light. As "art" displaces labour, the woman disappears behind her image. Even the title, by punning on the materialist parallel between cellophane and celluloid, makes the woman disappear.

Rimmer's films are filled with images of women. They seem, at first glance, to be almost synonymous with "the image" which is subjected to formal experiments, the classic example being *Variations on a Cellophane Wrapper*. And yet, one can also find a discourse on and about images of women, as well as an implicit critique of gender codes in their deployment. The more recent films may even be regarded as engaging with violence against women as a technology of language and representation. Like the slogan quoted above, though, the films tread a crooked path through feminist concerns, precisely because they are so often double-edged.[47] The work is remarkable in the preoccupation with women and the proliferation of images of women apprehended with an unsettling directness.

Bricolage is in a sense the recovery of the woman who is so cruelly violated and annihilated in *Variations*. An equally abstract image is gradually integrated, clarified, and resolved into a black-and-white image of a woman who appears to be advertising a cleaning product by sliding a piece of glass – one half clear, one half dirty – in front of her face. Her steady gaze through the glass at the camera is in direct contrast to the abrupt curtailment of the woman's look in *Variations*. A woman's voice repeats, "Plus ça change, plus c'est la même chose."

Without going so far as to say that *Bricolage* is the "corrected" version of *Variations*, other crucial elements of *Bricolage* suggest a real change in Rimmer's representation of women. The use of advertising imagery and the return of the gaze are key features, which recur in *As Seen on TV*, *Local Knowledge*, and *Black Cat White Cat*. By using shots clearly marked as commercial, the image is already exploited before Rimmer gets to it. His treatment is then a treatment of the image in its context. A good example of this is the women in colour-tests who appear in *Local Knowledge* and *Black Cat White Cat*. In the latter film, they serve as powerful signs of the gender codes of Chinese TV. Likewise, the "Toni Twins" in *As Seen on TV*, two women advertising a hair product who seem to float across the screen in Rimmer's video-manipulation of the original image, represent a 1960s representation of women.

All of these women look back at the viewer, and even if their address was originally that of the sales pitch, in their new contexts, their gaze is a challenge. It upsets the inertness of the material image, subjected again and again to formal manipulation, and becomes the sign of human presence. The Toni Twins also wipe off a piece of glass standing between them and the camera, and although the solarization of the image almost obscures their faces at times, their look still cuts through the many layers of aesthetic and historical mediation. Women remain identified with the image in Rimmer's films, as their faces and bodies become abstract patterns and formal movements through repetition, but in the formalization process, they also become the sign of "content" resisting that aestheticization – signs of dis-content.

Men also appear in the films, but their bodies are rarely the subject of intensive repetition and analysis, with the important exception of the naked man having an epileptic fit in *As Seen on TV*. However, privileged by the double framing and ominous electronic music (in contrast to the pop muzak of the rest of the film), this image evokes anxiety rather than objectification. The crisis of the film consists of the Toni Twins' endless gestures of walking, turning, entering, wiping, smiling, etc., as if they could never stop, as if they were trapped in those inane gestures for eternity. The doubling of the woman makes the play of looks very vivid, as at first one looks screen-right while the other looks at the camera. When they look at each other, the erotics of the image are strangely intensified, and when they both turn to the camera, the viewer is seduced in a way directly contrary to the daunting image of the naked man. Looking at him is a confrontation with alienation, fear, and mortal flesh. He represents the anxiety that the women seem to have caused through the soothing seduction of commercial media.

An earlier film, *Fracture* (1973), investigates the gendering of narrative codes. It is one of the only instances in which Rimmer uses his own footage – Super-8 blown up to 16mm – rather than found footage of women. Two series of shots are intercut. In one, a woman with a baby in a forest appears to fear something or someone approaching; in the other, a man in a cabin appears to open the door to leave. The latter series is somewhat obscure as the man's body is shot "too close," and yet that obscurity intensifies the sense of his bulk as well as the suspense. The woman exhibits the protective instincts of an animal mother, and her worried posture and expression enable us to read the other image as male and as threatening. Her look screen-right and his movement toward screen-left are spatial codes that narrativize two sequences which might in fact have nothing to do with each other.

The incorporation of the nuclear family within Rimmer's fracturing of narrative form is another example of the way in which a formal experiment acquires deep resonance through strategically chosen imagery. By alluding to a narrative of threatened innocence, he returns, through his own 1970s footage, to D.W. Griffith's early imbrication of narrative and social codes. The impression of continuity between the parallel series of images is only achieved through a scenario in which an active male discourse threatens a passive female one and the security of the family provides the stakes of the game. By the end of the ten-minute film the woman has returned to her sitting position, but there is no closure. Nothing has happened, but the sense of anticipation and suspense does not fade, suggesting again that the scenario is more permanent than its brief appearance in this film.

45

While narrativity tends to be generally downplayed in Rimmer's fragmented style of montage, in the later films an Eisensteinian aesthetic of juxtaposition and collision persists within the formal technique. Dialectical meanings emerge from the evocative imagery, meanings that continually circulate around women and violence. In *Local Knowledge* a collection of images linking an animated bull (like a cave painting) writhing with spears in its back, a mustached man (possibly a toreador), and a hunter provide a counterpoint to the Chinese woman's graceful, peaceful dance. Images of execution, surveillance, and explosions punctuate the film, and a rare example of a recognizable figure – the evangelist/cult leader Claire Prophet – intones the impending apocalypse in synch sound. Her reference to the darkness moving against the light is taken up in Rimmer's landscape photography, but another image later in the film gives it an ambiguous political implication: a documentary (not found) image of a graffiti slogan, "Reflet de nuit." Among the people who pass by the wall bearing this message are women who stop to look at the camera, women who begin and end the sequence. The extremely melancholy soundtrack links this section to the previous one of surveillance and crowds.

At another point in *Local Knowledge* a woman's legs are intercut with the image of fish mentioned above as an image suggestive of "the unconscious." After three quick shots of the legs, a man shooting a rifle appears briefly. Then Rimmer cuts back to the legs and the camera pans up the woman's body. The woman, perhaps from the 1940s, reclining slightly to show off her legs, turns and returns the gaze before we cut back to the fish. In one sense, the sequence is a dangerous flirtation with clichés of female sexuality, but with that look back at the camera, the woman reclaims her legs and extracts herself from the montage to reveal the fish and the gun as mere symbols. The sequence itself becomes a fragment of language rendered harmless in its deconstruction, but suggestive of impending violence.

While *Local Knowledge* is riddled with images of violence, *Bricolage* may be the film that engages most systematically with violence against women. It opens with a primitive audio-visual machine like a kinetoscope in which a woman's head appears in a small opening while a hand turns the crank, and a female voice intermittently squeaks "Hello." A graphic target is superimposed on the aperture. The suggestion of containment recurs in the final sequence in which a graphic white rectangle is superimposed on the image that eventually "becomes" the woman holding the piece of glass described above. Until we see this glass, it is graphically represented as a frame sliding back and forth in front of the woman's face.

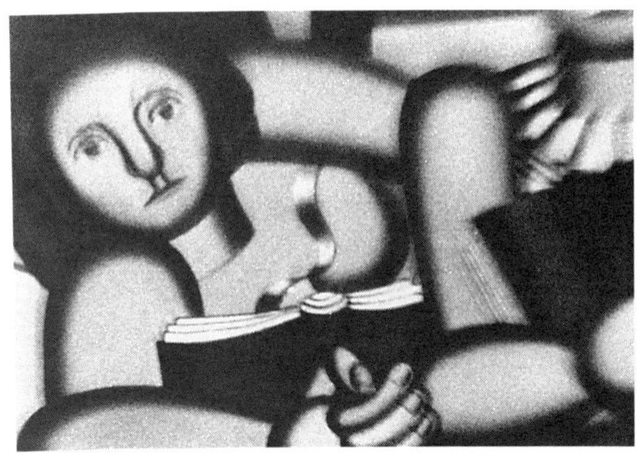

Beaubourg Boogie Woogie 1991

Local Knowledge 1992

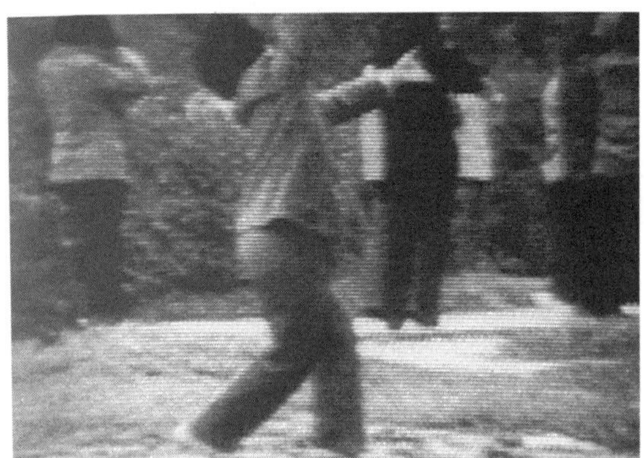

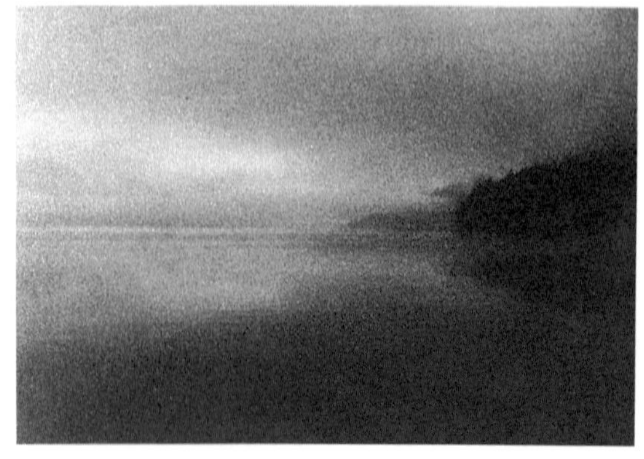

Local Knowledge 1992

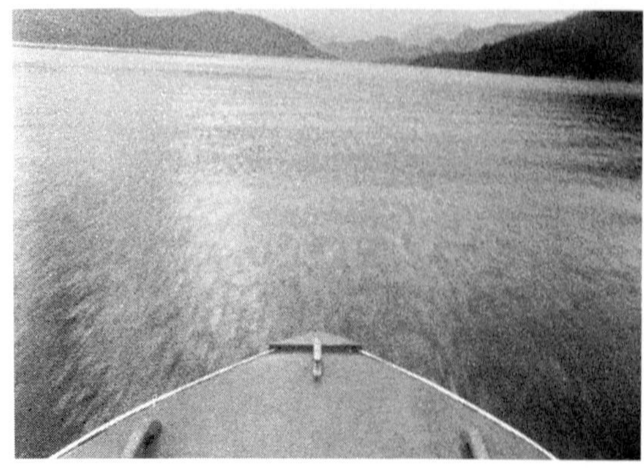

The white rectangle is also linked to a very specific site of violence when it is super-imposed on a window smashed by a hammer. The smashing action is part of a highly melodramatic and narratively coded scenario of male aggression, repeated twelve times, complete with escalating soundtrack.

Connecting these and other images of *Bricolage* is a black-and-white suggestion of a brick wall crumbling to reveal the woman advertising the cleaning product. She seems to be behind this wall, contained in the film like the woman in the box. Fragments of the phrase "Plus ça change ...," repeated monotonously by a woman's voice, accompany the wall image as well as the woman herself, whose lips move slightly out of synch with the phrase. It would do a disservice to the film to say that the phrase refers to women's role in the media, because referentiality is, as always, outside the scope of the film. And yet, the "bricolage" of the film is clearly more than a merely formal exercise, incorporating as it does a series of defamiliarized gender stereotypes from a range of historical sources. "Nothing changes" in this history upon which *Bricolage* comments without entering, retaining that distance of aloof observation that also characterizes the representation of landscape and culture in Rimmer's films.

It is precisely in the way images are offered up without commentary and with-out resolution that Rimmer disturbs and provokes. In *As Seen on TV* a colour image of a belly dancer mechanically performing in a boxlike set is distorted in such a way that only her face and her bare stomach can be clearly discerned. This is one of the women who never return the gaze; like the Chinese woman, she appears to be in a trancelike state. A man beside her seems to be touching her nipples with a pointer, as if she were the topic of a lecture. The violence of the scene consists in its repetition; the man's insistence and the woman's passivity are looped in an end-less activity of exhibitionism and aggression that incorporates the spectator as the man's interlocutor. Whatever the original footage may have looked like, Rimmer reduces it to a form of gender coding in a technology of address.

The point of this reading of gender in Rimmer's films is neither to accuse Rimmer of "incorrectness" nor to claim the films for a feminist agenda. It is rather to draw attention to the central place of gender in his analysis of representation, for it is spoken, written, and visual language with which the films are ultimately preoc-cupied. To this extent the work remains within a modernist paradigm of reflexivity and self-referentiality. Increasingly, though, this paradigm is not simply one of film language and representation, but in encompassing video, becomes a technolo-gy of representation. Language lessons, cave paintings, military weather forecasts, and all the other fragments of representation and pieces of language that come together in *Local Knowledge* become parts of a technology which is not inert, and is certainly not harmless.

Teresa de Lauretis argues that "violence is not simply 'in' language or 'in' representation, but it is also thereby en-gendered."[48] Her claim that "for the female subject, finally, gender marks the limit of deconstruction, the rocky bed (so to speak) of the 'abyss of meaning' "[49] is remarkably borne out in Rimmer's films. The exercises in form continually circulate around the female image which brings, in de Lauretis's words, "the sense of a certain weight of the object in semiosis, an overdetermination wrought into the work of the sign by the real."[50] Rimmer's representation of women may be anchored in a "pop" aesthetic of political ambiguity, but by linking that imagery with a violence of and in representation, he transcends the image itself and situates it within a technology of representation in which women are systematically violated.

Conclusion: The Work of Film

[F]or contemporary man the representation of reality by the film is incomparably more significant than that of the painter, since it offers, precisely because of the thoroughgoing permeation of reality with mechanical equipment, an aspect of reality which is free of all equipment. And that is what one is entitled to ask from a work of art.[51]

At one point in *Local Knowledge*, in shades of bright yellow and deep brown shadow, the cameraman (Rimmer) runs tight circles around a rock that remains centre-frame in close-up, medium close-up, and extreme close-up. The low angle is shaky, catching glimpses of the surrounding landscape, and the imagery has been made distinctly "painterly" through video effects. A rock on a mudflat is basically transformed into a van Gogh wheat field in a two-minute-long shot. Inserted into a rapidly paced section of the film loaded with images of violence, literal and metaphoric, this scene is relieving, despite the sound of footsteps and heavy breathing. It seems to anchor the body to its environment in a centred composition in which the very idea of a centre is banalized as a conveniently placed rock. The futility and physicality of the exercise, and the glimpses of Rimmer's shadow in the remote setting, make the sequence a grimly ironic comment on the labour of artmaking.

Two more recent films, *Beaubourg Boogie Woogie* (1991) and *Divine Mannequin*, also incorporate a strong sense of energy and labour linked to the act of filmmaking. Edited to the rhythm of a boogie woogie piano score, *Beaubourg Boogie Woogie* takes the viewer on a whirlwind tour of a gallery in the Centre Pompidou in Paris. Works by Picasso, Leger, Matisse, Magritte, Duchamp, and others are "collaged" in the rapid rhythms and camera movements which allow only fragmentary glimpses of the pieces. The film is transgressive in its disrespect for the conventions of contemplation demanded by wall art. The jazz soundtrack, however, evokes the dynamics of folk art that inspired much of the art in question, and its repetitions, along with the fast-paced editing, also reanimate the machine aesthetic of the period. The film may appear to subordinate high modernism to the popular cultural musical form that governs the film, and yet it shares a great deal with the work that it photographs in the tendency toward abstraction and its reflexivity. It ends with a long contemplative shot fixed on the sky framed by Beaubourg-district buildings, a very filmic image, offering a sigh of relief outside the gallery.

Beaubourg Boogie Woogie challenges the rarefied atmosphere of "art," not by bringing the paintings to life, but by parodying the gallery setting of the art. The energetic pace of the film represents a technologized, highly distracted gallery patron: a tourist perhaps, but also a physical presence. The tensions between formalist aesthetics and lived, experiential reality inform Rimmer's use of found footage, his use of structural techniques, and also the role of his own body in his films. *Divine Mannequin*, for example, is "grounded" in the image of Rimmer's own running feet, seen from above. A technologized self is indeed constant throughout this body of work in which the filmmaker himself never appears. It is his gaze which is represented in the persistently fixed camera position, a look that is not "all-perceiving" but materially and spatially linked to the filmmaker's body.

Blaine Allan has suggested that the video effects of *Divine Mannequin* approximate the "hand-made" qualities of film animation and a "corresponding restoration of traditional values to the high-tech artist working in film and video."[52] The document that accompanies the installation (a found text) endows it with a peculiarly mystical character, possibly of Buddhist origin, and at the same time identifies it obliquely with the male body.[53]

The auratic unities of traditional artmaking and art-viewing can still be found in Rimmer's work, but always at a distance, held at arm's length from the highly coded and technologized interaction with the world. If, for Walter Benjamin, "that which withers in the age of mechanical reproduction is the aura of the work of art,"[54] Rimmer relocates that aura as the trace of something sacred and vaguely erotic lingering just beyond the reach of mechanically reproduced imagery. The films are neither "modern" nor "postmodern," but tread a careful path between such categories. The work remains a far cry from George Kuchar's scatological and omnipresent self-representation, eschewing Kuchar's kitsch for a more reflective, and by contrast, modernist, aesthetic.

From the expressionistic mysticism of *Migration* (1969), in which Rimmer links Brakhagian camera-work to symbols of pop mysticism, to the sophisticated collage of landscape photography, found footage, and electronic sound which is *Local Knowledge*, Rimmer's films embrace technology as a mode of awareness. The subject of perception is immersed in a world that is increasingly recognized as gendered, as ethnically diverse, as historical, and as dangerous. As artistic subjectivity is pushed further and further into the shadowed recesses of the apparatuses of representation, so it seems is the "aura" of the work of art. Its passing is not mourned but configured as the trace of history, like the people of the past looking through the photographic residue of time.

Most of Rimmer's nonexperimental films are concerned with artistic practice as cultural activity that extends well beyond the art gallery. His most recent video, *Perestroyka* (1992), conforms closely enough to documentary convention that it may even find TV airtime. The interviews that make up *Perestroyka* are primarily with artists, filmmakers, musicians, and critics who address the difficulties of artistic activity in the Soviet past and the Russian present. *Al Neil: A Portrait* (1979), another fairly straightforward documentary, is a portrait of an experimental British Columbia artist/musician/poet/"character." Even in the experimental films, there is an ongoing interrogation of the relation of film to "art" in its gallery sense, an ambivalence concerning mechanical reproduction as artistic practice and experience.

The internal frames of so much of the imagery in *As Seen on TV* and *Local Knowledge* turn the film screen into a metaphorical TV screen. The digitalization of the imagery, however, tends to foreground the signifier, pushing signification into the background, a process more akin to the visual arts than to television. Such ambivalence points to the common tendencies of both television and wall art to enclose and confine "reality." Along with the windows and sheets of glass noted in *Bricolage*, Blaine Allan has noted that in the video installation version of *Divine Mannequin*, the stacked monitors look like windows through which we perceive the highly abstracted imagery, windows like those in *Real Italian Pizza* and the *Canadian Pacific* films.[55] In *Local Knowledge* and *Bricolage* white graphics superimposed on the image further equate the tendency towards enclosure with targets, "writing" the square or circular frame as a zone of desire and aggression.

All of these practices make literal the transformation of the real which takes place in framing. But reality does not become "auratic" through this framing; as it becomes desirable and commodified, it becomes language. Landscape and people, especially women, are potentially caught up in a technology of desire from which the eye of the camera escapes outside the frame. But as the eye of the camera and the "I" of the filmmaker become increasingly linked in a physical sense, the metaphysical/transcendental inscription of subjectivity is relegated to convention. Technology may insist on its perpetuation, but the living, breathing body of the filmmaker intrudes on its sovereignty. Those who are seen, on the other hand, on the other side of the apparatus, are freed from the technology of desire, and are allowed to return the gaze.

In this process, the imagery with which Rimmer works takes on an increasingly indexical relationship with its various sources, becoming "content," and recovering its signifieds. Insofar as the recurrence of West Coast horizons within his work constitutes a discourse of familiarity and emplacement, Rimmer is a "Canadian" filmmaker, not by virtue of a national aesthetic, but through a politics of location. Environmental issues may not be addressed any more literally than are feminist issues, and yet in *Local Knowledge*, at least, one feels obliquely the encroachment of destructive technology on a familiar landscape.

Black Cat White Cat closes with a stunning sequence in which the structural gaze, as the representation of determining consciousness, is quite literally relinquished. It begins with the camera positioned at the opposite end of Tiananmen Square from the entrance to the Forbidden City, a scene familiar to Western viewers from Bertolucci's *The Last Emperor* (1987). In the foreground of the shot, Chinese tourists, many of them sporting cameras, look at some "sight" hidden below the elevated camera angle, glancing up occasionally in the direction of the camera. The shot is held for some time, the dark interior of the distant palace mirroring the invisible camera in a structure similar to *Real Italian Pizza*, although the discomfort of some of the tourists aware of being watched makes it an even more panopticonic gaze. And then the camera pans slowly to the right, revealing a huge crowd gathered around, staring at the camera and its operator. As the multitude of curious tourists' faces unfolds with the camera movement, the centre of that movement, the filmmaker, becomes overwhelmed as the object of their gaze. We never see what they see because technology remains the province of individualized perception and the representation of subjectivity, and yet the cloak of invisibility has been penetrated. The game is up and the subject dethroned, simply by meeting the gaze of other people.

CONCORDIA UNIVERSITY, MONTREAL

Acknowledgements

I would like to thank David Rimmer, Peter Rist, Dave Douglas, Michael Gregory, and the Canadian Filmmakers Distribution Centre for their assistance in researching this essay.

1. Paul Mann, *The Theory-Death of the Avant-Garde* (Indiana: Indiana University Press, 1991), 40.

2. See Paul Arthur, "No More Causes? The International Film Congress," *The Independent* 12, no. 8 (October 1989): 22–26. That issue of *The Independent* also includes an open letter to the Experimental Film Congress from a group of filmmakers challenging its premises, and a response by Bart Testa as a member of the congress executive. See my essay "Will the Reel Avant-Garde Please Stand Up?" *Fuse* 13, no. 1–2 (Fall 1989): 37–43. See also Manhola Dargis, "The Brood," The Village Voice, 20 June 1989, 92.

3. P. Adams Sitney, *Visionary Film: The American Avant-Garde 1943–1978* (New York: Oxford University Press, 1979), 370.

4. The metaphysical connotations were developed mainly by Annette Michelson, "Toward Snow," 1971; rpt. in *The Avant-Garde Film: A Reader of Theory and Criticism*, ed. P. Adams Sitney (New York: New York University Press, 1978), 172–83; and Hollis Frampton, *Circles of Confusion: Film/Photography/Video, Texts 1968–1980* (Rochester, n.y.: Visual Studies Workshop Press, 1983).

5. Stephen Heath, "Repetition Time: Notes around 'Structural/Materialist Film,' " in *Questions of Cinema* (Bloomington: Indiana University Press, 1981), 165–75; Peter Gidal, *Materialist Film* (New York: Routledge, 1989); Malcolm Le Grice, *Abstract Film and Beyond* (London: Studio Vista, 1977).

6. Paul Arthur, "The Last of the Machine?: Avant-Garde Film since 1966," *Millennium Film Journal*, no. 16–18 (1986): 81.

7. Aside from Sitney, whose *Visionary Film* is subtitled "The American Avant-Garde 1943–1978," David James also deals extensively with structural film in a chapter called "Pure Film" in his *Allegories of Cinema: American Film in the 60s* (Princeton, n.j.: Princeton University Press, 1989). Neither mentions David Rimmer.

8. This is especially true of Al Razutis's essay for the Vancouver Art Gallery retrospective, "David Rimmer: A Critical Analysis," 1980; rpt. in *Take Two: A Tribute to Film in Canada*, ed. Seth Feldman (Toronto: Irwin, 1984), 275–86. For an appreciation of the "synaesthetic" properties of the films to 1971 which prioritizes "feelings" over content, see "David Rimmer: A Critical Collage," compiled by Joyce Nelson, in *Canadian Film Reader*, ed. Seth Feldman and Joyce Nelson (Toronto: Peter Martin Associates, 1977), 338–44.

9. A fourth paradigm, that of historiography, has already been developed in my article "Reproduction and Repetition of History: David Rimmer's Found Footage," *CineAction!*, no. 16 (Spring 1989): 52–58.

10. "The End of Avant-Garde Film" is the title of an article by Fred Camper in *Millenium Film Journal*, no. 16–18 (Fall 1986–Winter 1987): 99–124, which ostensibly inspired the organization of the 1989 International Experimental Film Congress. The open letter to the Congress signed by seventy-six filmmakers concludes, "The Avant-Garde is dead. Long live the avant-garde" (*The Independent* 12, no. 8 [October 1989]: 24).

11. Mann claims that the avant-garde "was condemned to death by its own idea of progress"

(Mann, 40). His obituary/historicization is as much of and for the discursive space surrounding adversarial art in postmodern culture as for the work itself, and is in this sense extremely pertinent to the situation of avant-garde film theory and criticism.

12. Frampton, 123.

13. Kirk Tougas, "Vancouver Letter," Take One 2, no. 11 (May–June 1970): 29.

14. Gaile McGregor, *The Wacousta Syndrome: Explorations in the Canadian Landscape* (Toronto: University of Toronto Press, 1985), 99. The name "Wacousta" derives from the title of an 1832 novel by John Richardson in which "a profound fear of nature often seems to override any other response" (McGregor, 7).

15. Bart Testa, *Spirit in the Landscape* (Toronto: Art Gallery of Ontario, 1989), 11.

16. Stephen Heath writes: "The disunity, the disjunction of 'structural/materialist film' is, exactly, the spectator" (Heath, 167).

17. Reproduced in *Vancouver: Art and Artists 1931–1983*, Exhibition Catalogue (Vancouver: Vancouver Art Gallery, 1983), 228.

18. Reproduced in *Vancouver: Art and Artists*, 230.

19. Scott Watson, "Terminal City: Place, Culture and the Regional Inflection," in *Vancouver: Art and Artists*, 226–55. Many visual artists also turned to the styles and iconography of the Northwest Coast native cultures, which are by and large absent from Rimmer's filmmaking, perhaps because they do not lend themselves to cinematic appropriation. It may not be stretching the landscape theme too far to see it reappear in *Media Wall*, an installation by Rimmer, Bill Fix, and Tom Shandel, which is also somewhat totemistic in concept. The ruins of television sets are banked in "mountains" and "pillars" against a gallery wall, as part of the 1969 *Electrical Connection* exhibition at Vancouver Art Gallery (photo of installation in *Vancouver: Art and Artists*, 186).

20. Scott Watson, "Art in the Fifties: Design, Leisure, and Painting in the Age of Anxiety," in *Vancouver: Art and Artists*, 97–98.

21. Blaine Allan, "David Rimmer's *Surfacing on the Thames*," Cine-tracts 3, no. 1 (Winter 1980): 58.

22. Michelson, 175. She goes on to cite Husserl as the philosophical source for her notion of horizons of perception.

23. Trinh T. Minh-ha, When the Moon Waxes Red: Representation, *Gender and Cultural Politics* (New York: Routledge, 1991), 71.

24. James Clifford, The Predicament of Culture: Twentieth Century Ethnography, Literature, and Art (Cambridge: Harvard University Press, 1988), 9.

25. Ibid., 9.

26. Heath claims that structural-materialist film is "anti-voyeuristic" (Heath, 19), but he fails to demonstrate either the means or the effects of such anti-voyeurism.

27. Dai Vaughan describes the distinctive sense of formal spontaneity characteristic of the Lumières' cinema in "Let There be Lumière," in *Early Cinema: Space, Frame, Narrative*, ed. Thomas Elsaesser (London: British Film Institute, 1990), 63–67.

28. Bart Testa, *Back and Forth: Early Cinema and the Avant-Garde*, (Toronto: Art Gallery of Ontario, 1992), 19. Testa lists other key examples of structural films using early found footage: Ken Jacobs, *Tom, Tom, the Piper's Son* (1969); Hollis Frampton, *Public Domain* (1972), *Gloria!* (1979), and *Cadenza #1* (1977–80); Ernie Gehr, *Eureka* (1974) and *History* (1974); Al Razutis, *Visual Essays: Origins of Film* (1973–84); and Malcolm Le Grice, *After Lumière* (1974) (Ibid., 36).

29. Ibid., 92.

30. Ibid., 94.

31. See my "Reproduction and Repetition of History," 56.

32. James Clifford, "Of Other Peoples: Beyond the 'Salvage Paradigm,' " in *Discussions in Contemporary Culture*, no. 1, ed. Hal Foster (Seattle: Bay Press, 1987), 121.

33. Noël Burch, "A Primitive Mode of Representation?" in Elsaesser, ed., Early Cinema, 220–27. See also Noël Burch, *Life to Those Shadows*, trans. and ed. Ben Brewster (Berkeley: University of California Press, 1990). See the debates anthologized in Elsaesser, ed, *Early Cinema*.

34. "Every description or interpretation that conceives itself as 'bringing culture into writing' moving from oral-discursive experience (the 'native's', the fieldworker's) to a written version of that experience (the ethnographic text) is enacting the structure of 'salvage'...." James Clifford, "On Ethnographic Allegory," in *Writing Culture: The Poetics and Politics of Ethnography*, ed. James Clifford and George E. Marcus (Berkeley: University of California Press, 1986), 113.

35. In the panopticonic institutionalized gaze of prison architecture, authority rests in centrality and invisibility; visibility becomes a form of submission as the gaze becomes a form of entrapment. Michel Foucault, *Discipline and Punish: The Birth of the Prison*, trans. Alan Sheridan (New York: Vintage Books, 1979), 195–230.

36. Roland Barthes, *Camera Lucida: Reflections on Photography*, trans. Richard Howard (New York: Hill and Wang, 1981), 34.

37. Ibid., 28.

38. Barthes defines the *noeme* "that-has-been": "[I]n Photography I can never deny that *the thing has been there*. There is a superimposition here: of reality and of the past" (ibid., 76).

39. Ibid., 82.

40. "[E]thnography's narrative of specific differences presupposes, and always refers to, an abstract plane of similarity" (Clifford, "On Ethnographic Allegory," 101).

41. Here I am obliquely alluding to Foucault's analysis of *Las Meninas* in order to indicate the tightly structured scenario of the empowered gaze which is reproduced in *Real Italian Pizza*. Michel Foucault, *The Order of Things: The Archeology of the Human Sciences* (New York: Vintage Books, 1973), 3–16.

42. Rimmer has identified the location as the Upper West Side, around 85th Street and Columbus. Rick Hancox claims to have spotted Rimmer himself eating pizza on the other side of the camera, suggesting a further breakdown of the voyeuristic set-up (Rick Hancox, "Short Films," *Cinema Canada*, 2d ser., no. 14 (June–July 1974): 58–60.

43. Trinh, 96.

44. Clifford Geertz, *Local Knowledge: Further Essays in Interpretive Anthropology* (N.p.: Basic Books, 1983), 6.

45. Clifford, *The Predicament of Culture*, 40.

46. Ibid., 94–95.

47. For a history of the "exclusively male subject-position" in the avant-garde, see Susan Suleiman, *Subversive Intent: Gender, Politics, and the Avant-Garde* (Cambridge: Harvard University Press, 1990), 21.

48. Teresa de Lauretis, *Technologies of Gender: Essays on Theory, Film and Fiction* (Bloomington: Indiana University Press, 1987), 42.

49. Ibid., 48.

50. Ibid., 41.

51. Walter Benjamin, "The Work of Art in the Age of Mechanical Reproduction," in Illuminations, trans. Harry Zohn (New York: Schocken Books, 1969), 234.

52. Blaine Allan, "Handmade, or David Rimmer's *Divine Mannequin*," Canadian Journal of Film Studies 2, no. 1 (1992): 66.

53. Blaine Allan has suggested that the text is "consistent with some accounts of the sacraments of Tantrism and Buddhist practice" although the source is unknown. It describes a female totem through which a religious man can "make love to a semidivine" (ibid., 72). *Divine Mannequin* was installed at Emily Carr College's Charles E. Scott Gallery in September 1988 in the form of three stacked monitors and a text tacked on the wall. According to Allan, "the column of images effectively becomes a body" (ibid., 69).

54. Benjamin, 221.

55. Allan, 70–71.

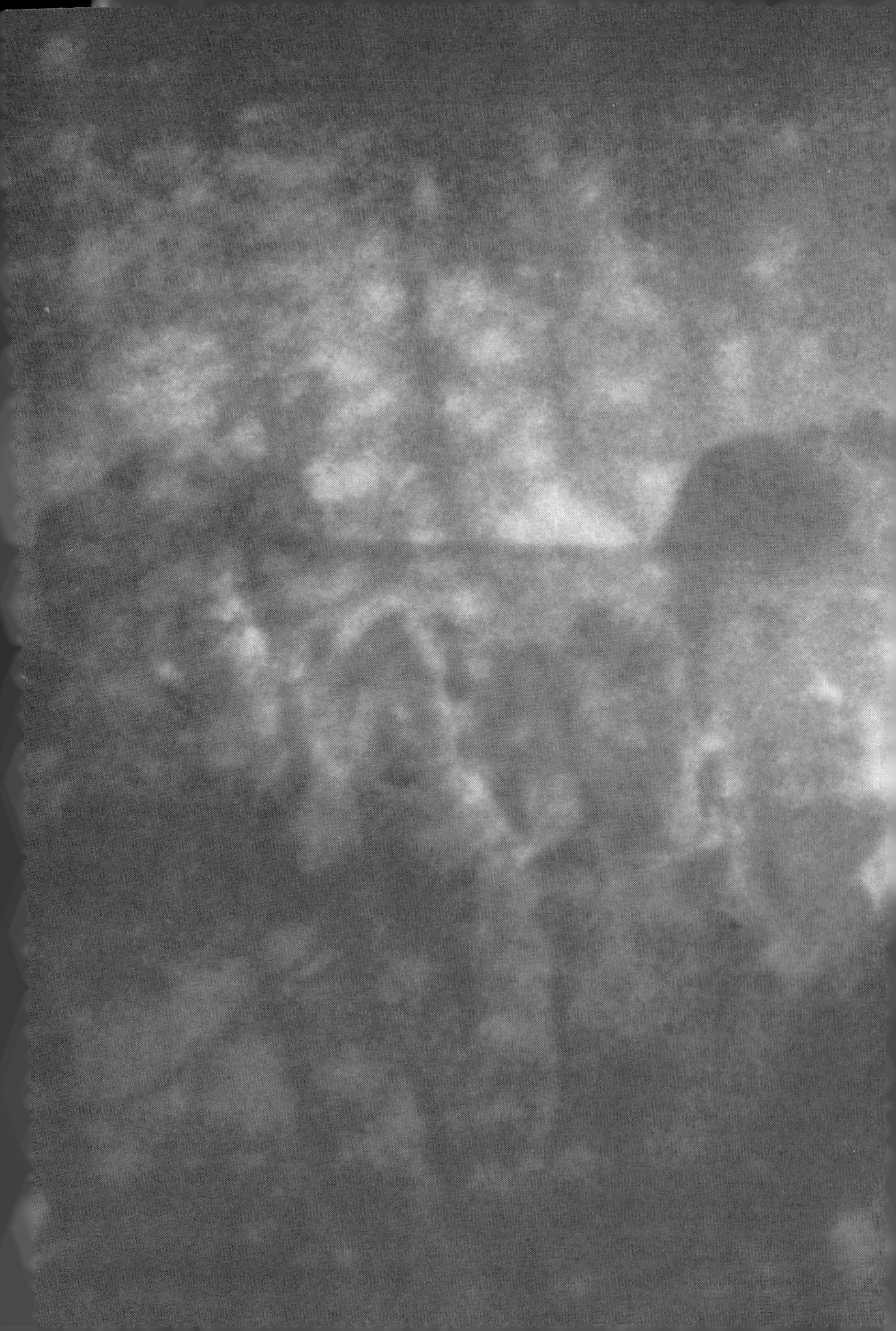

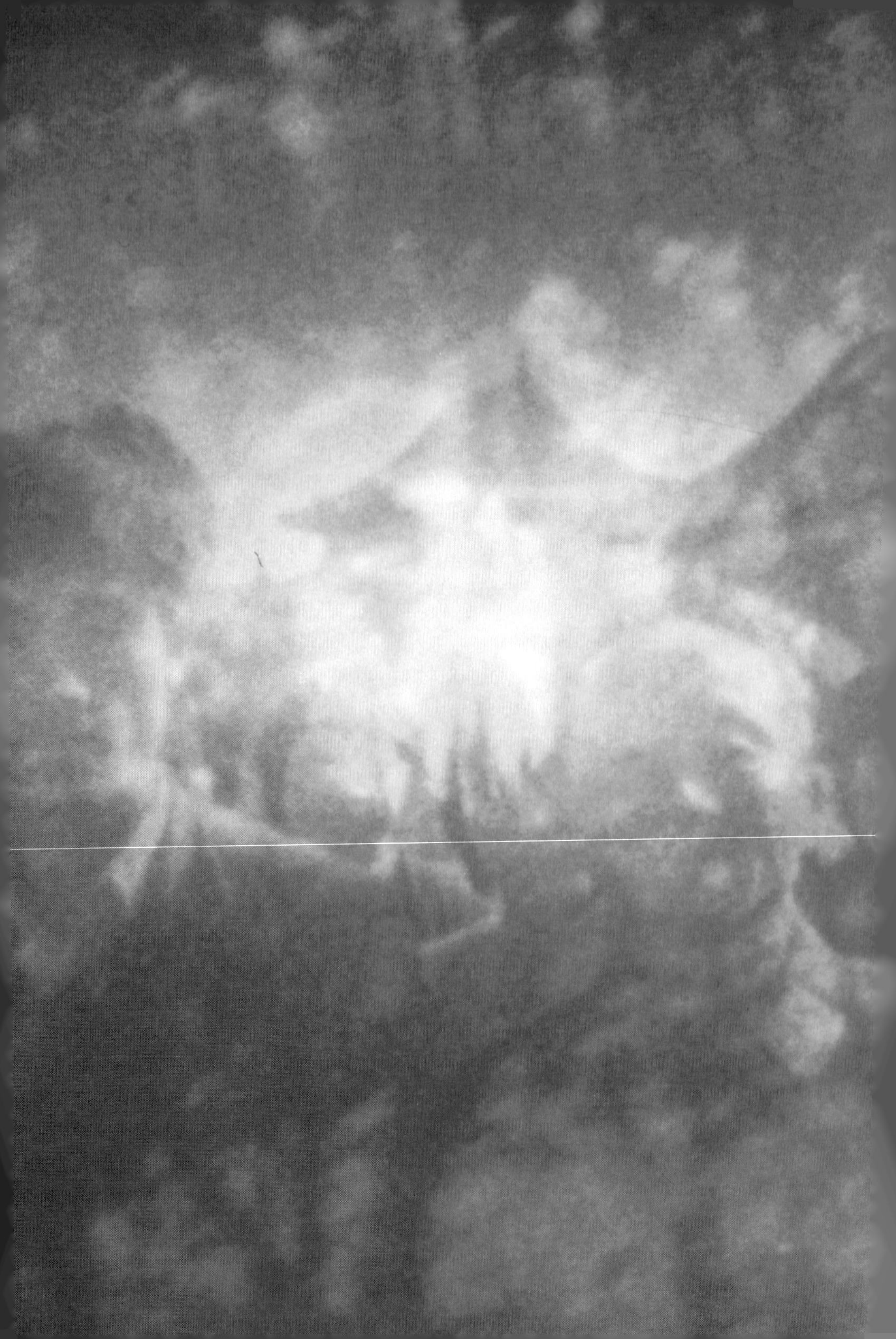

Filmography

Head/End. 1967, 2 min., col.

Knowplace. 1967.

West Coast. 1967–present, 2 hours +, col. and b&w, silent and sound.
An open-ended and extended portrait of a group of people who collectively own a piece of land on the West Coast, north of Vancouver. It is made primarily for this group but is occasionally shown outside this context.

Square Inch Field. 1968, 13 min., col.

Landscape. 1969, 8 min., col., silent.

Migration. 1969, 11 min., col.

Blue Movie. 1970, 6 min., col., silent.

The Dance. 1970, 5 min., b&w.

Surfacing on the Thames. 1970, 9 min., col., silent.

Treefall. 1970, 5 min., b&w, silent.

Variations on a Cellophane Wrapper. 1970, 8.5 min., col.

Real Italian Pizza. 1971, 13 min., col.

Seashore. 1971, 11 min., b&w, silent.

Fracture. 1973, 10 min., col., silent.

Watching for the Queen. 1973, 11 min., b&w, silent.

Canadian Pacific. 1974, 9 min., col., silent.

Canadian Pacific II. 1975, 9 min., col., silent.

Shades of Red. 1977, 40 min., col.

Al Neil: A Portrait. 1979, 40 min., col.

Narrows Inlet. 1980, 10 min., col., silent.

Bricolage. 1984, 11 min., col.

Along the Road to Altamira. 1986, 20 min., col.

As Seen on TV. 1986, 14 min., col., also on video.

Black Cat White Cat It's a Good Cat if It Catches the Mouse. 1989, 35 min., col.

Divine Mannequin. 1989, 7 min., col.

Beaubourg Boogie Woogie. 1991, 5 min., col.

Local Knowledge. 1992, 33 min., col.

(all films have sound unless otherwise noted)

Videography

Show of Numbers. 1975, b&w, video installation.

Box Cars. 1975, 4 min., col.

Hello. 1978, 7 min., b&w.

Solo from Chaos. 1983, 10 min., col.

Bach Duet. 1983, 8 min., col., two-monitor piece.

Sisyphus. 1984, 22 min., col.

Steal the Thunder. 1986, 10 min., col.

As Seen on TV. 1986, 14 min., col., also on film.

Roadshow. 1987, 21 min., col.

Divine Mannequin. 1989, col., video installation.

Perestroyka. 1992, 85 min. col.

A Guide to the Film Literature

by Kathryn Elder

with the assistance of
Susan Oxtoby and
Gayathry Sethumadhavan

1969

1001
Reif, Tony. "Letter from Vancouver." *Take One* 2, no. 2
(October 1969): 26.
Reviews the Vancouver Art Gallery benefit screening for the Intermedia Film
Cooperative. Rimmer's *Square Inch Field* (1968) and *Migration* (1969) are among the
highlights. They bring out the interconnectedness of all things: the latter achieves
this through the associative use of imagery while the former relies on startling visual
effects and rhythms.

1002
Schroeder, Andreas. "Movies: Producers Rate Top Honors." *Province*
(Vancouver), 12 September 1969, 33.
Reviews films by Rimmer, Al Razutis, and Keith Rodan in the Vancouver Art Gallery
benefit show. Describes *Migration* (1969) as a "re-discovery of the energy, menace or
beauty of things one may have passed many times before."

1003
Townsend, Charlotte. "And the Camera Betrays the Hand and Eye."
Vancouver Sun, 12 September 1969, 29.
Reviews the Vancouver Art Gallery benefit screening for Intermedia Film Cooperative.
Says Rimmer avoids the excesses of other underground filmmakers. Praises *Landscape*
(1969) for its visual beauty and *Migration* (1969) for bringing forth the "pulse and
vitality of nature in the raw."

1970

1004
Daniels, Edgar. "The Ann Arbor Film Festival: An Applause of Films."
New Cinema Review 1, no. 3 (1970): 20–26.
Praises *Surfacing on the Thames* (1970) for its painterly quality but also reports that the
audience did not share the reviewer's enthusiasm.

1005
Paquet, Andre. "Qu'est-ce que le cinema canadien?" Trans. Penni Jacques.
Artscanada, no. 142–143 (April 1970): 3–6.
An overview of the problems besetting Canadian film production, followed by a
description of some positive regional initiatives. Lists Rimmer among a new generation
of Vancouver artists whose distinctiveness rests in the intensely personal and contemplative quality of their work.

1006
Schroeder, Andreas. "Films: Simple Genius." *Province* (Vancouver),
31 July 1970, 6.
Reviews *Variations on a Cellophane Wrapper* (1970), focusing on Rimmer's ability to create
"a barrage of metaphor" about the environment with simple source material and modest
expenditure.

1007
Tougas, Kirk. "Vancouver Letter." *Take One* 2, no. 11 (May–June 1970): 29.
Reports on the new vitality of West Coast filmmakers working with the short film, a for-
mat which allows them to refine ideas in successive works. Using Rimmer's recent films
as examples, comments on the progression from *Landscape* (1969), *The Dance* (1970), and
Surfacing on the Thames (1970) to *Variations on a Cellophane Wrapper* (1970), explaining
that the limited modulation of activity in the first three is opened up in the last film.

1008
Youngblood, Gene. "The New Canadian Cinema: Images from the Age of
Paradox." *Artscanada*, no. 142–143 (April 1970): 7–13.
Encountering Rimmer's work is called the highlight of the author's introduction to new
Canadian film. *Square Inch Field* (1968) and *Migration* (1969) are excellent examples of
"synaesthetic cinema," a form that transcends cultural and linguistic boundaries because
its focus is the unity underlying all things. Praises *Square Inch Field* because it "surveys
the micro-macro universe as contained in the mind of man." Says *Surfacing on the Thames*
(1970) is the ultimate metaphysical movie as it "confronts empirically the illusions of
space and time in the cinema."

1971

1009
Curtis, David. "Opticals – Film as Film and Found Footage."
In *Experimental Cinema: A Fifty Year Evolution*, 140–46.
London: Studio Vista, 1971.
Briefly describes filmmakers who are reworking imagery with rephotography. Rimmer's
refilming and use of lap dissolves in *Surfacing on the Thames* (1970) result in a tightly
structured film.

1972

1010

Gilbert, Gerry. "An Evening of Dave Rimmer's Films." In *Form and Structure in Recent Film*, ed. Dennis Wheeler, n. pag. Exhibition Catalogue. Vancouver: Vancouver Art Gallery and Talon Books, 1972.

Includes some biographical information about Rimmer and the author's personal responses to ten of Rimmer's films.

1011

Greenspun, Roger. "The Films of David Rimmer." *New York Times*, 26 February 1972, 18.

Reviews Rimmer's program at New York's Film Forum. *Seashore* (1971) and *The Dance* (1970) are "ghostly evocations of lost energy" in contrast to the stillness of *Surfacing on the Thames* (1970), while the jaunty mood of *Real Italian Pizza* (1971) really captures the essence of city life.

1012

———. "Quick — Who Are David Rimmer and James Herbert?" *New York Times*, 8 October 1972, sec. 2, p. 17.

Introduces the filmmakers as artists who should be better known to New York audiences. Both share an interest in the dissolution of the image but Rimmer's films are less grounded in dramatic content and possess greater wit.

1013

"In View." *Art and Artists* 7, no. 9 (December 1972): 8–9.

Lists Rimmer among the filmmakers included in the Vancouver Art Gallery exhibition *Structural Cinema*, organized by Dennis Wheeler.

1014

Le Grice, Malcolm. "Thoughts on Recent Underground Film." *Afterimage* (London) 4 (Autumn 1972): 78–95.

Offers an alternative to P. Adams Sitney's definition of structural film because it excludes the work of many filmmakers, Rimmer among them.

1015

Melnyk, L. "Experimental Films ... 'The Flawless Pattern of Rotation.' " *Queen's Journal* (Kingston), 29 September 1972, 8.

Variations on a Cellophane Wrapper (1970) is shown at Queen's University in a program organized by the Agnes Etherington Gallery. Praises the film's formal unity and compares the imagery to "the sea's rhythmic fall and swell."

1016
Moritz, William. "Film Books: Three Books on Experimental Cinema."
Film Quarterly 25, no. 4 (Summer 1972): 31–34.
Sees the strength of David Curtis's *Experimental Film: A Fifty Year Evolution* (see entry
1009) in the overview it provides of North American and European filmmaking. Among
the examples cited is Curtis's comparison of optical printing activity and reference to
Rimmer.

1017
Nordstrom, Kristina. "Film: Celebrations of Life and Death."
Village Voice (New York), 6 April 1972, 79.
Reviews a series of Rimmer shows at New York's Film Forum. Describes the different
forms of movement that are the subject of Rimmer's scrutiny, the techniques he uses to
alter the rhythms in the parent footage, and the painterly affinities that result. *Variations
on a Cellophane Wrapper* (1970) and *Real Italian Pizza* (1971) receive the most attention,
with the colour patterns in the former likened to abstraction and the combination of
human anecdote and formalism in the latter to the work of Edward Hopper.

1018
———. "The Films of David Rimmer." *Film Library Quarterly* 5, no. 3
(Summer 1972): 28–31, 41.
Reprint of entry 1017.

1973

1019
DuCane, John. "The Festival of Light and Time Continues." *Time Out*, 7
September 1973.
Reports on the highlights of the final days of London's Festival of Independent/
Underground Film. Rimmer's name appears in the concluding paragraph with other
filmmakers collectively referred to as "The Rest."

1020
"Exhibition of Contemporary Canadian Art to Be Held in Paris."
Cinema Canada, 2d ser., no. 8 (June–July 1973): 9.
Lists Rimmer among Canadian filmmakers in the *Canada Trajectoires 73* exhibition at
the Musee d'Art Moderne de la Ville de Paris.

1021
Klepac, Walter. "Art: Films by David Rimmer." *Guerilla* 3, no. 24
(March 1973): M2
Reviews an Art Gallery of Ontario screening of Rimmer's films, calling them "lucid" and
"self-contained," akin to "a set of musical variations." Suggests Rimmer's use of a single
sequence rather than a plurality of images in his later films accounts for their stronger
audience appeal because his "inventive variations" of ordinary images give people a clear-
er picture of the process of human perception. Describes the action in *Variations on a
Cellophane Wrapper* (1970) as a "progressive reduction" with "a logical sequence" and a
"wry recapitulation of the development from representational to abstract painting ... in
exclusively cinematic terms."

1022
Koller, George Csaba. "Filmpeople, Filmpeople, Filmpeople."
Cinema Canada, 2d ser., no. 7 (April–May 1973): 15.
Notes Rimmer's presence at an Art Gallery of Ontario screening of *Real Italian Pizza*
(1971) and *West Coast* (1967–) prior to his departure for a European tour with shows
scheduled in Moscow, West Berlin, London, Amsterdam, Oslo, and Milan.

1023
Le Grice, Malcolm. "Vision." *Studio International* 185, no. 952
(February 1973): 52.
Announces Rimmer's availability for shows in Britain. Calls him and Jack Chambers
the most interesting filmmakers to emerge from Canada since Michael Snow and Joyce
Wieland and notes Gene Youngblood's high praise for *Surfacing on the Thames* (1970)
(see entry 1008).

1024
———. "Vision." *Studio International* 185, no. 953 (March 1973): 104.
Lists Rimmer among the filmmakers who must be offended at Jonas Mekas's obituary
notice for Jerome Hill in the 7 December 1972 issue of *Village Voice* because Mekas
implies that the great creative period in American filmmaking has ended and the next
stage should be one of evaluation and preservation.

1025
Nicolson, Annabel. "Canadada Fragments." *Art and Artists* 8, no. 1
(April 1973): 28–33.
Reflections of a British filmmaker who toured North America with a package of structural
films from the London Film Cooperative. Comments that Rimmer is one of the few
Canadian filmmakers who is aware of film as process, citing the loop printing in *Seashore*
(1971), the time lapses in *Real Italian Pizza* (1971) and *Landscape* (1969), and the
refilming in *Surfacing on the Thames* (1970).

1026
Paquet, Andre. "Cineastes: Les espaces visuels ou les savants du 24 images seconde." In *Canada Trajectoires 73*, n. pag. Exhibition Catalogue. Montreal: Editions Mediart, 1973.
Attributes the exuberance of North American independent filmmakers to the individualism characteristic of the culture and suggests their innovative work is the best artistic weapon to enliven perceptions dulled by Hollywood. Briefly notes regional differences in Canada, citing Rimmer's contemplative approach as indicative of the freshness of West Coast filmmaking.

1027
————. "Cinema experimental: Les espaces visuels ou les savants du 24 images seconde." *Cinema Quebec* 3, no. 1 (September 1973): 33–35.
Reprint of entry 1026.

1974

1028
"David Rimmer." *In Personal Film: Content and Context*, ed. Tony Rief and Kirk Tougas. Vancouver: Intermedia Press, 1974.
Rimmer's entry for the series (organized by the Pacific Cinematheque) contains excerpts from the commentary of Roger Greenspun (see entry 1012), Kirk Tougas (see entry 1007), and Kristina Nordstrom (see entry 1017) on three films: *Variations on a Cellophane Wrapper* (1970), *Seashore* (1971), and *Real Italian Pizza* (1971).

1029
Edwards, Natalie. "Moving Art." *Cinema Canada*, 2d ser., no. 13 (April–May 1974): 54–55.
Reviews some of the work in the National Gallery of Canada's Filmmakers Series, a selection of thirty short films designed to give a capsule view of independent filmmaking since 1967. *Migration* (1969), *Blue Movie* (1970), and *Real Italian Pizza* (1971) appear in the individual program descriptions.

1030
Freyer, Ellen. "Formalist Cinema: Artistic Suicide in the Avant-Garde." *Velvet Light Trap* 13 (Fall 1974): 47–49.
Rimmer's name appears in this negative assessment of American structural filmmaking which dismisses the work because human experience is no longer the focal point of artistic concern.

1031

Gale, Peggy. "The National Gallery's Canadian Filmmakers Series: Canadian Artists as Filmmakers." *Artmagazine* 6, no. 19 (Fall 1974): 28.
Reviews the National Gallery of Canada's Filmmakers Series. Describes *Real Italian Pizza* (1971) as "a stop-and-go montage of store front activity."

1032

Hancox, Rick. "Short Films." *Cinema Canada*, 2d ser., no. 14 (June–July 1974): 58–60.
Reviews the National Gallery of Canada's Filmmakers Series. Notes the inclusion of *Migration* (1969), *Blue Movie* (1970), and *Real Italian Pizza* (1971). The behaviour of the antiheroes in the landscape of the latter is especially appealing because of the temporal paradoxes Rimmer has created for them through rephotography, fixed framing, and the high-angle camera shots.

1033

Ibranyi-Kiss, A. "Filmmaking West Coast Style: Jack Darcus." *Cinema Canada*, 2d ser., no. 13 (April–May 1974): 42–45.
Cites Rimmer as one of a group of West Coast filmmakers who has developed a body of work with a personal viewpoint.

1976

1034

Edwards, Natalie. "It's Film All Right, but Is It Art?" *Cinema Canada*, 3d ser., no. 26 (March 1976): 18–20.
Reviews a two-part package of Canadian experimental films assembled by the National Gallery of Canada and distributed by the Canadian Filmmakers' Distribution Centre. Included are Rimmer's *Fracture* (1973), *Watching for the Queen* (1973), and *Canadian Pacific* (1974). Says he is one of the most exciting artists in North America today and praises the films for drawing viewers' attention to the subtleties of perception.

1035

Eizykan, Claudine. "La distribution des ecarts." In *La jouissance – cinema*, 292–96. Paris: Union Generale d'Editions, 1976.
Describes the strategies filmmakers use to highlight interaction between film frames. Rimmer renders movement almost imperceptible in *Surfacing on the Thames* (1970), *Watching for the Queen* (1973), and *A Narrative Film* [*Fracture* 1973], thereby isolating and enhancing action and human gesture. He achieves the same effect in *Real Italian Pizza* (1971) but with different means.

1036
Gould, Michael. "The Artist-Inventor." Chap. in *Surrealism and the Cinema*.
London: Tantivy, 1976.
Says minimalism and surrealism share a common vision to expand human consciousness
at all levels by bringing the spectator out of an insular world into metaphysical awareness. The former attempts this by emptying an artwork of nonessential elements so that
its basic nature is perceived in conceptual revelations. Film has a minimalist tradition
dating back to the work of Edison where simple human gestures were extended over time
and became the sole subject of the work. Rimmer's *The Dance* (1970), which possesses
a "crazy absurdity," has a precursor in Rene Clair's *Entre'acte* (1924), where the action of
a washerwoman climbing a flight of stairs is repeated.

1977

1037
Beattie, Eleanor. "Rimmer, David." In *A Handbook of Canadian Film*,
163–64. 2d ed. Toronto: Peter Martin Associates, 1977.
Praises Rimmer's ability to take stock footage and make fresh transformations of film
clichés, giving as examples *Variations on a Cellophane Wrapper* (1970), *The Dance* (1970),
and *Surfacing on the Thames* (1970). Includes filmography and seven-item bibliography.

1038
Birnie, Ian, Tony Reif, and Jean-Pierre Bastien. "Independent Views."
Cinema Canada, no. 38–39 (June–July 1977): 45–49.
Fracture (1973) and *Canadian Pacific* (1974) are included in a three-part series of Canadian
independent films coordinated by the Art Gallery of Ontario and the National Film Board
of Canada and distributed by the Canadian Filmmakers' Distribution Centre.
The Vancouver films evoke a sense of the timeless through formal means. Rimmer's aesthetic approach is described in a quotation from Robert Fothergill: "taking some part of a
recorded action, he distills it to an abstract pattern then slowly allows its contents to seep
back in like an epiphany."

1039
Ibranyi-Kiss, A. "Filmmaking West Coast Style: Jack Darcus."
In *Canadian Film Reader*, ed. Seth Feldman and Joyce Nelson, 268–73.
Toronto: Peter Martin Associates, 1977.
Reprint of entry 1033.

1040

Le Grice, Malcolm. "Current Developments." Chap. in *Abstract Film and Beyond.*
Great Britain: Studio Vista, 1977.
Surveys international filmmaking activity. Cites *Surfacing on the Thames* (1970), which
makes use of refilming material from the screen in a controlled manner, as one of the
most interesting examples of image transformation.

1041

Nelson, Joyce, comp. "David Rimmer: A Critical Collage." In *Canadian Film
Reader*, ed. Seth Feldman and Joyce Nelson, 338–44. Toronto: Peter Martin
Associates, 1977.
Series of positive remarks about Rimmer's films excerpted from the commentary of Kirk
Tougas (see entry 1007), Tony Reif (see entry 1001), Kristina Nordstrom (see entry 1017),
Roger Greenspun (see entry 1012), and Walter Klepac (see entry 1021).

1042

Siegel, Lois. "Experimental Films, Ignored." Letter. *Cinema Canada*, no. 41
(October 1977): 5.
Expresses concern about the decision to drop the Experimental Film category from the
Canadian Film Awards. Rimmer, along with other Canadians, is known internationally
for this type of filmmaking.

1043

Youngblood, Gene. "The New Canadian Cinema: Images from the Age of
Paradox." In *Canadian Film Reader*, ed. Seth Feldman and Joyce Nelson,
323–32. Toronto: Peter Martin Associates, 1977.
Reprint of entry 1008.

1978

1044

Bassan, Raphael. "Experiences canadiennes." *Cinema different*, no. 21–22
(June 1978): 12–13.
Reviews a National Gallery of Canada touring package of experimental films following its
July screening at the Canadian Cultural Centre in Paris. Calls Rimmer's *Blue Movie*
(1970) a semi-abstract symphony which plays with colour variations in the waves.

1045
Koller, George Csaba. "David Rimmer: Honesty of Vision." *Cinema Canada*, no. 44 (February 1978): 18–21.
A biographical sketch in which Rimmer reveals the creative impulse behind his work and the modest production techniques he uses. His early films were shaped by an interaction with performance events and he has maintained his interest in environmental sculpture, painting, and sound. He calls himself an "artist" who is working with film.

1046
————. "Le cinema experimental." In *Les cinemas canadiens*, ed. Pierre Lherminier, 61–70. Montreal: La Cinematheque Quebecoise, 1978.
A cross-country assessment of filmmaking activity that omits the West Coast but concludes with a quotation by Rimmer about the positive attitudes of his students: their primary interest is in exploring the artistic potential of film rather than acquiring skills for the industry.

1047
Reif, Tony, and Kirk Tougas. "Le cinema de la cote ouest." In *Les cinemas canadiens*, ed. Pierre Lherminier, 47–60. Montreal: La Cinematheque Quebecoise, 1978.
Gives a brief history of the Vancouver film community and profiles individual filmmakers. Describes the evolution in Rimmer's work from the rapid camera movement and editing in *Square Inch Field* (1968) and *Migration* (1969) to the contemplation of quiet and subtle movements in *Canadian Pacific* (1974) and *Fracture* (1973).

1048
Thoms, Albie. "The International Avant Garde Film Festival: 1973." Chap. in *Polemics for a New Cinema*. Sydney: Wild and Woolley, 1978.
Highlights interesting work at this London event. Rimmer's name appears in a list of filmmakers in attendance.

1979

1049
Ward, Melinda. "Independent Film in Minneapolis/St. Paul." *Millennium Film Journal*, no. 4–5 (Summer–Fall 1979): 144–52.
An overview of local exhibition facilities. Rimmer's name appears in a list of nationally recognized filmmakers invited to screen work at the Walker Art Center in the first season in its new building.

1980

1050
Allen [sic], Blaine. "David Rimmer's *Surfacing on the Thames.*" *Cine-tracts* 3,
no. 1 (Winter 1980): 56–61.
Attempts to give the film an aesthetic context but finds its complexities exceed the narrow
boundaries imposed by the conflicting notions of structural and experimental film as
defined by P. Adams Sitney and Peter Wollen. Supports this position by pointing out the
film's simultaneous concerns with realism and illusionism, mathematical precision and
dramatic structure, two- and three-dimensional space, still and apparent movement, as
well as surface texture and colour.

1051
Razutis, Al. "David Rimmer: A Critical Analysis." In *David Rimmer Film*,
n. pag. Exhibition Catalogue. Vancouver: Vancouver Art Gallery, 1980.
Gives Rimmer's work a regional context with a description of a diverse West Coast artistic
community that cut across national borders and so brought Canadian filmmakers into
contact with American aesthetics. Especially influential for Rimmer were Stan Brakhage's
concept of a personal vision and the notion of the frame, rather than the shot, as the basic
unit of filmic construction, and Bruce Conner's manipulation of stock footage into tightly
structured social critiques. Distinguishes Rimmer's work from the British structuralist-
materialist school by its complexity of filmic design and poetic content, and in a detailed
analysis of each film, indicates the conceptual problem Rimmer is exploring. Includes
filmography and career highlights.

1981

1052
Brown, Colin. "David Rimmer: Re-Fusing the Contradictions."
Parachute, no. 22 (Spring 1981): 48–49.
Reviews Rimmer's retrospective at the Vancouver Art Gallery where eleven of his eighteen films were screened. Admires his ability to make "intelligent and poetic" films that
stand up over time and display a human element in spite of the formal issues underpin-
ning them. Notes a similarity of subject matter in *Migration* (1969) and *Narrows Inlet*
(1980), compares the step-by-step explorations in *Variations on a Cellophane Wrapper*
(1970), *Surfacing on the Thames* (1970), *Real Italian Pizza* (1971), and *Seashore* (1971) to
Gertrude Stein's methodical inquiries into language, comments on the dramatic strategies of the long take and parallel montage developed in *Watching for the Queen* (1973) and
Fracture (1973), and praises *Al Neil: A Portrait* (1979) for its "quiet personal style" which
allows the man to emerge from the legend. Encourages Rimmer to continue the use of
chance elements like the fog and waves in *Narrows Inlet* because they pose visual challenges to his highly developed technique.

1053
Feldman, Seth. "Film: The Path Not Taken." *Canadian Forum*,
November 1981, 39–40.
Rimmer's international reputation is noted in this discussion of what distinguishes
experimental filmmaking from narrative feature filmmaking.

1054
Lamb, Jamie. " 'My Films Are Difficult to Watch.' " *Vancouver Sun*,
8 January 1981, C1.
The retrospective of Rimmer's films at the Vancouver Art Gallery evokes mixed reactions
from visitors. In response, Rimmer likens his interest in frame-to-frame relations and
perception to the painter's interest in the impact of different strokes and the other
material components of his art.

1055
Nelson, Joyce. "Shorts: *Al Neil: A Portrait*." *Cinema Canada*, no. 73
(April 1981): 47.
Characterizes Rimmer's early films as metaphysical and cerebral because they possess a
wholeness that transcends dualities and invites quiet contemplation. *Al Neil: A Portrait*
(1979), in contrast, has a rough texture that personifies the man the film portrays but it
rewards the empathetic viewer who experiences both the depths of Neil's despair and the
celebration of his life.

1056
Perry, Art. "Entertainment: Rimmer Turns Film to Art." *Province*
(Vancouver), 7 January 1981, A8.
Reviews Rimmer's retrospective at the Vancouver Art Gallery. Applies Al Razutis's
remarks about the films' minimalist qualities (see entry 1051) to the discipline and
restraint evidenced in *Variations on a Cellophane Wrapper* (1970), *Seashore* (1971), and
Al Neil: A Portrait (1979).

1982

1057
Elder, R. Bruce. "Redefining Experimental Film: Postmodernist Practice
in Canada." *Parachute*, no. 27 (Summer 1982): 4–9.
Excerpt from entry 1067.

1058

————. "'All Things in Their Times.'" *Cine-tracts* 5, no. 1 (Summer–Fall
1982): 39–45.
Concludes an article from an earlier issue of *Cine-tracts* (3, no. 1) about the postmodernist
attributes of Michael Snow's *Back and Forth* (1968) and the artist's pioneering role in
making this the distinctive feature of much Canadian experimental filmmaking. In
Rimmer's *Surfacing on the Thames* (1970) this takes the form of balancing the illusionistic
and nonillusionistic aspects of film. Extending the boat's movement through rephotography makes evident frame-to-frame relations and elements of the picture plane that are
responsible for the three-dimensional representation in the stock footage.

1059

Feldman, Seth. "Making It: Business as (Un)usual." *Cinema Canada*,
no. 81 (February 1982): 22–23.
An assessment of contemporary Canadian experimental film that lists Rimmer as one
of its leading figures.

1060

Larouche, Michel. "Films experimentaux." *Parachute*, no. 28 (September–
October 1982): 36–37.
Migration (1969) and *The Dance* (1970) appear in a three-day program of eighteen films
at Montreal's Vehicule Art, selected to represent the aesthetic concerns of independent
filmmakers over the past twenty years. Associates Rimmer's work with the structural
movement, briefly describes the optical transformations in the two films, and notes their
hypnotic appeal.

1983

1061

"Artists' Biographies: David Rimmer." In *Vancouver: Art and Artists* 1931–1983,
422. Exhibition Catalogue. Vancouver: Vancouver Art Gallery, 1983.
Includes a selective list of exhibitions, festival screenings, and institutional film sales.
Among the purchasers are the National Gallery of Canada, the Museum of Modern Art,
and the British Film Institute.

1062

Elder, Bruce. "The Canadian Avant-Garde." In *Canadian Images: Festival of
Canadian Film*, 27–29. Festival Catalogue. Peterborough: Canadian Images, 1983.
Canadian Pacific II (1975), *Seashore* (1971), *Surfacing on the Thames* (1970), and *Narrows
Inlet* (1980) are included in a nine-part program of Canadian experimental films that sur-
veys explorations of the properties of the photographic image.

1063
Razutis, Al. "Rediscovering Lost History: Vancouver Avant-Garde Cinema
1960–69." In *Vancouver: Art and Artists* 1931–1983, 160–73. Exhibition
Catalogue. Vancouver: Vancouver Art Gallery, 1983.
Contrasts the vibrancy of the multimedia work that flourished in the 1960s with the minimalism of structuralism, describes the individuals and organizations who supported this
"synaesthetic" cinema, and profiles some of the filmmakers. Notes that Rimmer was
attracted to both performance-based and structural filmmaking: *Treefall* (1970) was part of
a dance performance, *Blue Movie* (1970) was projected on a geodesic dome, and *Landscape*
(1969) was conceived as a "wall-framing" installation, while *Head/End* (1967), *Square
Inch Field* (1968), and *Migration* (1968) highlighted montage and compositional patterns.
Credits Rimmer with redefining structural film with works like *Variations on a Cellophane
Wrapper* (1970), *Surfacing on the Thames* (1970), and *Seashore* (1971). In these, he achieved
a balance between styles by using stock footage that related metaphorically to the conceptual problems he was exploring.

1064
Razutis, Al, and Tony Reif. "Critical Perspectives on Vancouver Avant-Garde
Cinema 1970–83." In *Vancouver: Art and Artists* 1931–1983, 286–99.
Exhibition Catalogue. Vancouver: Vancouver Art Gallery, 1983.
Comments on the plurality of work that characterized the decade and describes as
significant trends the "video-film-hybrids," which challenged the minimalism of structural film and reflected a regional predisposition to "iconoclastic practice," and the interest
in a socially relevant avant-garde. The profile on Rimmer points out elements common to
several films: the issue of viewership in *Real Italian Pizza* (1971), *Watching for the Queen*
(1973), *Canadian Pacific* (1974), and *Canadian Pacific II* (1975), and the narratives developed from simple stock footage sequences in *Fracture* (1973) and *Watching for the Queen*
(1973). Attributes Rimmer's abandonment of structural filmmaking in the mid 1970s to
the limits inherent in his working method and concludes by contrasting his return to formal concerns in *Narrows Inlet* (1980) with the subjectivity of *Al Neil: A Portrait* (1979).

1065
Wees, William C. "The Apparatus and the Avant-Garde." *Cinema Canada*,
no. 97 (June 1983), Special Supplement: 41–46.
Rimmer's optical printing is cited along with techniques used by other filmmakers as a
valid analysis of the cinematic apparatus in this response to theorists who are wary of formal innovations that do not foreground ideological issues.

1984

1066
Banning, Kass. "Re/Vision: Reconsidering the British and Canadian
Avant-Garde Cinemas." In *A Commonwealth*, ed. Lori Keating and
Kass Banning, n. pag. Exhibition Catalogue. Toronto: Funnel, 1984.
The purpose of the series is to challenge assumptions about British avant-garde films
being concerned exclusively with theory and radical politics and Canadian avant-garde
films with aesthetics and personal expression. Rimmer's *Variations on a Cellophane
Wrapper* (1970) is a film that combines politics and personal expression since women's
labour is one of its themes.

1067
Elder, R. Bruce. "Image: Representation and Object: The Photographic
Image in Canadian Avant-Garde Film." In *Take Two: A Tribute to Film in
Canada*, ed. Seth Feldman, 246–63. Toronto: Irwin, 1984.
A catalogue essay written for the 1982 *OKanada* Berlin art exhibition and reprinted here
in its entirety. Proposes that Canadian experimental filmmakers are forerunners in the
development of postmodernist forms of cinema, using as evidence their interest in the
photographic characteristics of the medium. Describes two aspects of Rimmer's films:
temporal paradox and framing. The contents of *Seashore* (1971), *The Dance* (1970),
Surfacing on the Thames (1970), and *Watching for the Queen* (1973) evoke nostalgia which
Rimmer counteracts by emphasizing the medium's physical properties like grain or the
frame-to-frame movement, thus highlighting the tension between presence and absence
that is characteristic of a photograph. The many references to the boundaries of the frame
in *Canadian Pacific* (1974) imply its control over perspective, and the dual projection of
Canadian Pacific and *Canadian Pacific II* (1975) alludes to the process of making the films.

1068
———. "Experiments: The Photographic Image." In *Festival of Festivals,
1984*, 156–64. Festival Catalogue. Toronto: Festival of Festivals, 1984.
Ten of Rimmer's films are included in a twenty-part program that considers Canadian
avant-garde filmmaking in the context of a realist tradition in Canadian art. Emphasizes
Rimmer's use of the optical printer as an analytical tool of photographic illusionism.

1069
Morris, Peter. "Rimmer, David." In *The Film Companion*, 256–57.
Toronto: Irwin, 1984.
Rimmer, next to Michael Snow, is perceived internationally as Canada's best-known film
artist. Comments on the dual nature of the films; their interest in the medium's structural properties is balanced by a meditation on film as a metaphor for perception. Includes
filmography and extensive bibliography.

1070

————. *"Surfacing on the Thames."* In *The Film Companion*, 286. Toronto: Irwin, 1984.

Calls this "elegant, austere" film one of Rimmer's major works and a key film in the tradition of Canadian experimental film. Includes a five-item bibliography.

1071

Razutis, Al. "David Rimmer: A Critical Analysis." In *Take Two: A Tribute to Film in Canada*, ed. Seth Feldman, 275–86. Toronto: Irwin, 1984.

Reprint of entry 1051.

1072

————. "Ménage à Trois: Contemporary Film Theory, New Narrative and the Avant-Garde." *OPSIS: The Canadian Journal of Avant-Garde and Political Cinema* 1, no. 1 (Spring 1984): 52–66.

Footnote 11 describes the film program accompanying the 1983 Vancouver conference, New Narrative Cinema and Future of Film Theory, as an inverted chronology of experimental film's progression towards "new narrative." Says Rimmer's work is the "Structuralist" and "Structuralist/Materialist" component.

1073

Testa, Bart. "Experimental Film: Its Past, Its Future." *Globe and Mail* (Toronto), 31 August 1984, E3.

Reports on the experimental film component of the Canadian retrospective at the 1984 Toronto Festival of Festivals. Describes *Surfacing on the Thames* (1970) and *Seashore* (1971) as the "most magical and precise" in the genre of Canadian landscape films.

1985

1074

Bendahan, Raphaël. "Experimental Cinema in Canada." *Vanguard* 14, no. 5–6 (Summer 1985): 18–21.

Remarks that young women filmmakers prefer narrative strategies over the formal and romantic traditions pioneered by Michael Snow and Rimmer, respectively. *Variations on a Cellophane Wrapper* (1970) and Snow's *One Second in Montreal* (1969) exemplify these older aesthetic movements and make clear what is shaping the work of younger filmmakers. Rimmer's permutations evoke a trancelike state which invites pleasure but denies insight into the filmmaking process, while Snow's use of visual imagery as data promotes an aggressive analysis of the medium but at the expense of human insight.

1986

1075
Elder, R. Bruce. "Experiments: The Photographic Image." In *Northern Lights: A Programmer's Guide to the Festival of Festivals Retrospective*, ed. Michael Sean Kiely, 87–103. Ottawa: Canadian Film Institute, 1986.
Reprint of entry 1068 with capsule summary of the theme and French translation of the program notes.

1076
Everett-Green, Robert. "Frames from beyond the Fringe." *Globe and Mail* (Toronto), 13 May 1986, d9.
Highlights interesting films at Experimental/streetwise, a two-hour, three-decade survey at the Rivoli Cafe during Toronto's Artweek. Describes Rimmer's manipulaton of advertising imagery in *As Seen on TV* (1986) as a "virtuosic repertoire of color-printing devices" and advises anyone going to the premiere of *Along the Road to Altamira* (1986) at the Art Gallery of Ontario to "bundle up against a very cool esthetic."

1077
———. "Art: Celluloid Experiments." *Globe and Mail* (Toronto), 6 September 1986, c13.
Reviews *As Seen on TV* (1986) and *Along the Road to Altamira* (1986) as part of the Canadian experimental film component at the 1986 Toronto Festival of Festivals. Prefers the former because of its virtuoso optical printing and, like the best of Rimmer's work, its ability "to forge an image template in the mind, something to endure after the actual images have been burnt away." The imagery in the second film is far less compelling by comparison.

1078
Freyer, Ellen. "Cinema formansta: Suicidio artistico dell'avantguardia." In *New American Cinema: Il cinema indipendente Americano degli anni sessanta*, ed. Adriano Arpa, 147–52. Torino: Festival of Internazaionale Cinema Giovani, 1986.
Italian reprint of entry 1030.

1079
Russell, Katie. "Festival Hits Home." NOW (Toronto), 28 August–3 September 1986, 23.
Reviews Rimmer's *Along the Road to Altamira* (1986) and *As Seen on TV* (1986) among the Canadian experimental films at the 1986 Toronto Festival of Festivals. The former "demonstrates the creative potential of travel footage" while the latter is "an implicit, agonizing, perspective on the institution of television."

1080

Sternberg, B. "On (Experimental) Film." *Cinema Canada*, no. 128
(March 1986): 56.
Notes Rimmer's participation in a panel discussion, "Avant-Garde Film Practise: Six
Views," part of the week-long celebrations to mark the opening of Vancouver's Pacific
CineCentre.

1081

————. "On (Experimental) Film." *Cinema Canada*, no. 130 (May 1986): 45.
Lists Rimmer among five filmmakers premiering new work in the Art Gallery of
Ontario's program Survey: '60s, '70s, '80s.

1987

1082

Allan, Blaine. "It's Not Finished Yet (Some Notes on Toronto Filmmaking)."
In *Toronto: A Play of History*, ed. Louise Dompierre, 83–92. Exhibition
Catalogue. Toronto: Power Plant, 1987.
Written to accompany four programs of experimental films made by Toronto-area
filmmakers between 1976 and 1986. Identifies two common themes: the search for an
artistic voice and the sense of personal dislocation. Says filmmaker Phil Hoffman
includes a brief "quotation" from Rimmer's *Watching for the Queen* (1973) in his *?O, Zoo!*
(The Making of a Fiction Film) (1986) as part of an acknowledgement to the Canadian documentary film tradition.

1083

Clandfield, David. "Animated Film and Experimental Film." Chap. in
Canadian Film. Toronto: Oxford University Press, 1987.
Short synopsis of Rimmer's career that links his films according to technique: *Variations
on a Cellophane Wrapper* (1970) and *Seashore* (1971) – film loops; *Surfacing on the Thames*
(1970) and *Watching for the Queen* (1973) – modulated collage sequences; and *Canadian
Pacific* (1974) and *Canadian Pacific II* (1975) – framing references.

1084

Insell, Maria. "En Garde: Echoes in the Museum of an Official Canadian
Avant-Garde." *Speed* 1, no. 1 (Spring 1987): 37–43.
Edited transcript of panelists' statements at the 1986 Cineworks seminar, "Avant-Garde
Film Practise: Six Views," one of several events to celebrate the organization's move into
new quarters. Participating with Rimmer were Michael Snow, Patricia Gruben, Joyce
Wieland, Ross McLaren, Lenore Coutts, and Al Razutis. Rimmer advocates less reliance
on verbal and written texts in experimental film and video, calling this practice an "obses-

sion with meaning and with words" that detracts from the intrinsic sensuous power of
the image and arises from "an erotic need to strip the image of its mystery."

1085

Kerr, Richard. "On (Experimental) Film." *Cinema Canada*, no. 145
(October 1987): 78–79.

A discussion about film education that lists Rimmer among the groundbreaking film
artists whose work should be part of the curriculum of Canadian universities.

1086

"Montage of Voices." *Millennium Film Journal*, no. 16–18 (Fall 1986–
Winter 1987): 250–73.

Excerpts from statements made by filmmakers who have shown work at Millennium.
Rimmer comments in a 1974 appearance that he has used editing in his silent films to
create visual patterns analogous to musical rhythms.

1087

Sternberg, B. "On (Experimental) Film." *Cinema Canada*, no. 142
(June 1987): 48.

Laments the exclusion of experimental films from critics' discussions of contemporary
Canadian art, citing Rimmer's *Bricolage* (1984) as an obvious example.

1988

1088

Brakhage, Stan. "Some Words on the North." *American Book Review* 10,
no. 2 (May–June 1988): 5, 18.

Describes the impetus for his program of Canadian experimental films The Aesthetic of
the North presented at the University of Colorado, at Boulder. He shares with the Group
of Seven a respect for the harshness of the natural landscape, quoting American poet
Charles Olson ("Nature? ... She'll kill you, given the chance!"), and believes their artistic
legacy has been carried forward by Canadian experimental filmmakers. Refers to
Rimmer's *Along the Road to Altamira* (1986) as a "peopleless travelogue through the
mind."

1089

Elder, R. Bruce. "Films, Experimental." In *Canadian Encyclopedia*, ed.
James H. Marsh. 2d ed. Edmonton: Hurtig, 1988.

Attributes the rapid growth of experimental film in the late 1960s to the appearance of
the postmodernist aesthetic, whose concern with photography and representation struck
a responsive chord in Canadians with an artistic commitment to representational art.

Groups films that explore the different properties of photographic representation into three categories: the landscape film, the diary film, and theme and variation films which often make use of optical printing. Lists *Real Italian Pizza* (1971), *Canadian Pacific* (1974), and *Canadian Pacific II* (1975) in the first group, and *Surfacing on the Thames* (1970) and *Watching for the Queen* (1973) in the third group.

1090
———. "Rimmer, David." In *Canadian Encyclopedia*, ed. James H. Marsh. 2d ed. Edmonton: Hurtig, 1988.
Emphasizes the common elements in Rimmer's work and that of the Toronto school of experimental filmmakers: Rimmer's films "are no less austere, have no more surface polish, and are no more contemplative ... and most are produced using rudimentary rather than advanced technologies." Characterizes Rimmer's films as "painstakingly careful examinations of how film constructs the illusion of movement, depth, continuity and audience presence at the situation depicted."

1091
Knight, Deborah. "Exquisite Nostalgia: Aesthetic Sensibility in the English-Canadian and Quebec Cinemas." *CineAction!*, no. 11 (Winter 1987–1988): 30–37.
Suggests that the Canadian documentary film tradition is responsible for a conflict in English-Canadian and Quebec feature films and experimental films between a desire for presence, documentation, and objectivity and a desire for representation, creativity, and illusion, which leaves the films without the sense of completion or the imagined unity of classical Hollywood cinema. The author defines this experience of difference as exquisite nostalgia, the tension between the temporal experience of the film and the absence of what it refers to, and describes the forms this takes. Rimmer's *Surfacing on the Thames* (1970), *Canadian Pacific* (1974), and *Canadian Pacific II* (1975) are cited in a list of films that express the tension by deferring pleasure – by extending the process through time.

1989

1092
Elder, R. Bruce. "All Things in Their Time: Michael Snow's *Back and Forth*." Chap. in *Image and Identity: Reflections on Canadian Film and Culture*. Kitchener: Wilfrid Laurier University; Toronto: Academy of Canadian Cinema, 1989.
Reprint of entry 1058 with minor additions and in the context of a detailed discussion regarding the origins of Canadian philosophical thought in Common Sense philosophy and Absolute Idealism and their impact on the evolution of the country's realist tradition in painting and film.

1093

———. "The Photographic Image in Canadian Avant-Garde Film." Chap.
in *Image and Identity: Reflections on Canadian Film and Culture*. Kitchener:
Wilfrid Laurier University; Toronto: Academy of Canadian Cinema, 1989.
Reprint of entry 1067 with minor additions and in the context of a detailed discussion
regarding the origins of Canadian philosophical thought in Common Sense philosophy
and Absolute Idealism and their role in the evolution of the country's realist tradition in
painting and film.

1094

Falsetto, Mario. "Recent Films from Canada." In *International Experimental
Film Congress*, ed. Kathryn Elder et al., 68–70. Exhibition Catalogue.
Toronto: Art Gallery of Ontario, 1989.
Rimmer's *As Seen on TV* (1986) is included in one of two programs devoted to Canadian
film. Although a part of Rimmer's ongoing investigation into the nature of the image, the
film is marked by a new "disturbing undercurrent."

1095

Insell, Maria. "En Garde: Desire in Ruins: Echoes in the Museum
of an Official Canadian Avant-Garde." *Independent Eye* 10, no. 3
(Summer 1989): 33–42.
Reprint of entry 1084.

1096

Punter, Jennie. "Entertainment: Experimental Cinema Series Opens
Tonight." *Whig-Standard* (Kingston), 18 October 1989: 32.
Announces Rimmer's appearance in the New Works Showcase Series at Kingston's
Princess Court Cinema and briefly comments on five films: *Bricolage* (1984), *As Seen on
TV* (1986), *Along the Road to Altamira* (1986), *Divine Mannequin* (1989), and *Black Cat
White Cat It's a Good Cat if It Catches the Mouse* (1989).

1097

Russell, Catherine. "Reproduction and Repetition of History:
David Rimmer's Found Footage." *CineAction!*, no. 16 (Spring 1989): 52–58.
Suggests that the critical frameworks developed by Al Razutis (see entry 1051) and Bruce
Elder (see entry 1067) for identifying postmodernist elements in Rimmer's work ignore
the impact of historical representation embodied in his manipulation of found footage.
Describes in detail the content of *Bricolage* (1984), *As Seen on TV* (1986), and *Along the
Road to Altamira* (1986), noting their paradoxes and contradictions and distinguishing
them from Rimmer's earlier films in their combination of altered sequences rather than
manipulations of a single action. Points out the cinematic references in *Bricolage*, and
comments on the unease that arises in *As Seen on TV* from the juxtaposition of the period

footage with the naked man masturbating as the private action represented in the latter
engenders a sense of voyeurism. Describes how Rimmer's mix of found footage and a
variety of on-site shooting in *Along the Road to Altamira* successfully captures the fragmented experience of the tourist whose ambition is to master the other culture through
observation.

1098

——. "Reviews: Film: Will the Reel Avant-Garde Please Stand Up?"
Fuse 13, no. 1–2 (Fall 1989): 37–43.
A critical assessment of the programming objectives of the 1989 International
Experimental Film Congress which observes that the many divisions that emerged along
the lines of age, gender, politics, and aesthetics were not always as clear-cut as partici-
pants claimed. Rimmer is one example: identified with the old, white, male avant-garde,
he demonstrates a cultural sensitivity in *Black Cat White Cat It's a Good Cat if It Catches
the Mouse* (1989) as he takes on the role of tourist in China.

1099

Testa, Bart. "A Presence in the Landscape." Chap. in *Spirit in the Landscape.*
Exhibition Catalogue. Toronto: Art Gallery of Ontario, 1989.
Canadian Pacific (1974), *Migration* (1969), and *Narrows Inlet* (1980) are in a five-part
series of Canadian experimental films that is thematically linked to the writings of
Northrop Frye and other cultural commentators about the representation of the landscape
in Canadian painting and literature. Rimmer's three films share a formal rigour but are
distinct in their response to the landscape. The iconography and composition of *Canadian
Pacific* reflect the "garrison mentality" or "boxed experience," where the landscape is perceived from the security of an enclosed space, while *Migration*'s frenetic style and elemen-
tal imagery of death and rebirth are the result of a direct confrontation with nature.
Narrows Inlet suggests a guarded acceptance of the natural world as it employs the
rhythms of the waves and fog to unveil a majestic panorama that maintains its mystery.

1990

1100

Czernis, Loretta. "Pourquoi est-ce que la bete est noire? A Brief Meditation
on Canadian Experimental Film." *Canadian Journal of Political and Social
Theory* 14, no. 1–3 (1990): 215–18.
Rimmer's *As Seen on TV* (1986) is on a list of Canadian works that challenge convention
and so fit the author's definition of experimental film in a rebuttal regarding the continu-
ing usefulness of the term. For the author, it means a "constellation of perspectives
which reflect Hollywood, and nationhood, thus revealing the more obscure membranes of
narrativity" and "opportunities to explore the fissures, crevices, wounds, and thresholds
of a so-called other and more dominant film dialect."

1101

Dorland, Michael. "'The Void Is Not So Bleak': Rhetoric and Structure in Canadian Experimental Film." *Canadian Journal of Political and Social Theory* 14, no. 1–3 (1990): 148–59.
Revised version of a 1988 presentation at the National Gallery of Canada. Accounts for the marginalization of Canadian experimental film by claiming that there has been no attempt to provide the work with an aesthetic framework, other than by foreign critics. Accepts Deborah Knight's concept of "exquisite nostalgia" (see entry 1091) and from it concludes that experimental film is only a variant of Canada's documentary tradition. Finds fault with both Bruce Elder's and Gaile McGregor's efforts to define unique elements in Canadian filmmaking and culture, although Dorland uses the former's "classic" text on the postmodernist aspirations of Canadian filmmakers (see entry 1067) to support his description of experimental filmmakers as documenting the transition from a naive to a self-conscious realism. He lists Rimmer's *Canadian Pacific* (1974) and *Canadian Pacific II* (1975) among the "classics" of the genre.

1102

Jonasson, Catherine, ed. *New Experiments*. Exhibition Catalogue. Toronto: Art Gallery of Ontario, 1990.
Eight Rimmer films are in a five-part program of Canadian experimental work at London's Canada House. Briefly describes the content of each, noting that they represent two of the three categories critics use to define his work: the media critique and the structural film. *Migration* (1969) is "atypical of Rimmer's oeuvre," *Canadian Pacific* (1974) is "the quintessential landscape film," *Narrows Inlet* (1980) is a "meditative" film that maintains a tension between "the panorama ... unveiled" and the "deep impenetrable space beyond," and *Black Cat White Cat It's a Good Cat if It Catches the Mouse* (1989) presents a China that is "full of contradictions and enormous potential for problems" as the people appear to be "tourists in their own land."

1992

1103

Allan, Blaine. "Handmade, or David Rimmer's *Divine Mannequin*." *Canadian Journal of Film Studies* 2, no. 1 (1992): 63–80.
Based on a presentation to the 1990 annual Conference of the Society for Animation Studies. Says the film defies the easy categorization of Rimmer's recent films, which can be grouped as media critiques or experimental travel documentaries. Contrary to the peacefulness implied by the title, the film exhibits an anxiety regarding the possibility of human intervention in artmaking in the video era. Identifies all the references to the human body in the film and shows how this theme is replicated in an installation also called *Divine Mannequin*. Rimmer arranged the images spatially on three stacked televi-

sion monitors with the runner's image at the bottom. He added an incomplete text he found on the Tantric Buddhist practice of hand-crafting wooden temple figures and placing children in them so that worshippers could experience a sense of realism in their sexual union with the divine. Notes Rimmer's analogy between these masters of illusion and contemporary film and videomakers.

1104
———. "David Rimmer's *Divine Mannequin*." In *Responses: In Honour of Peter Harcourt*, ed. Blaine Allan et al., 2–8. Kingston: Responsibility Press, 1992.
Edited version of entry 1103.

1105
Testa, Bart. "Early Episodes in the Career of the Gaze: Scanning the Primitive Tableau." Chap. in *Back and Forth: Early Cinema and the Avant-Garde*. Toronto: Art Gallery of Ontario, 1992.
A critical assessment of the new movements in film historicism which examine the cultural, economic, and social environments in which early cinema evolved and posit pedagogical links between it and the avant-garde. Discusses Rimmer's *Seashore* (1971) in a section about the relation of cinematic perspective and narrative to the voyeurism of Edison's minimally staged reproductions and the visual instability of the Lumières' single-shot panoramic documentaries which also contained controlled movements within the frame. Rimmer exposes the fragility of cinematic perspective by juxtaposing symmetrical but opposing repetitions of the same footage. The first section induces a contemplative engagement with the image which is abruptly disrupted with the cutting in of its reversal. Further distortions occur through editing, superimpositions, and optical printing.

1993

1106
Bordwell, David, and Kristin Thompson. "Mise-en-Scene in Space and Time." In *Film Art: An Introduction*, 163–72. 4th ed. New York: McGraw-Hill, 1993.
Cites *Watching for the Queen* (1973) as one example of the impact of static composition on the viewer's attention to subtle changes within a shot.

This bibliography is part of an ongoing series about Canadian experimental filmmakers. The author thanks the Ontario Arts Council and York University Libraries for their support.

Film Title Index

Blue Movie
1010, 1011, 1017, 1018,
1029, 1032, 1041, 1044,
1045, 1063, 1068, 1075

Bricolage
1087, 1090, 1096, 1097,
1102, 1103

Canadian Pacific
1034, 1038, 1045, 1047,
1051, 1057, 1064, 1067,
1068, 10671, 1075, 1083,
1089, 1091, 1092, 1099,
1101, 1102, 1103, 1104

Canadian Pacific II
1051, 1057, 1062, 1064,
1067, 1068, 1071, 1075,
1083, 1089, 1091, 1093,
1101, 1103, 1104

Commercial
1010

The Dance
1007, 1008, 1010, 1011,
1012, 1017, 1018, 1036,
1037, 1041, 1043, 1045,
1047, 1050, 1051, 1057,
1058, 1060, 1063, 1067,
1068, 1071, 1075, 1092,
1093

Divine Mannequin
1096, 1102, 1103, 1104

Fracture
1034, 1035, 1038, 1045,
1047, 1051, 1052, 1054,
1068, 1071, 1072, 1075,
1103

Head/End
1063

Landscape
1003, 1007, 1025, 1041,
1051, 1071

Migration
1001, 1002, 1003, 1008,
1010, 1011, 1017, 1018,
1021, 1026, 1027, 1029,
1032, 1041, 1043, 1045,
1047, 1051, 1052, 1060,
1061, 1063, 1068, 1071,
1075, 1099, 1102, 1103

Narrows Inlet
1052, 1062, 1064, 1090,
1099, 1102

Real Italian Pizza
1010, 1011, 1012, 1017,
1018, 1022, 1025, 1026,
1027, 1028, 1029, 1031,
1032, 1035, 1041, 1045,
1047, 1051, 1052, 1064,
1071, 1072, 1089, 1103

Seashore
1010, 1011, 1017, 1018,
1025, 1028, 1041, 1045,
1047, 1051, 1052, 1056,
1057, 1062, 1063, 1067,
1068, 1071, 1073, 1075,
1083, 1090, 1093, 1103,
1105

Square Inch Field
1001, 1008, 1010, 1011,
1017, 1018, 1021, 1041,
1043, 1045, 1047, 1051,
1061, 1063, 1071, 1103

Surfacing on the Thames
1004, 1007, 1008, 1009,
1010, 1011, 1012, 1017,
1018, 1023, 1025, 1026,
1027, 1035, 1037, 1039,
1041, 1043, 1045, 1050,
1051, 1052, 1057, 1058,

1062, 1063, 1067, 1068,
10670, 1071, 1072, 1073,
1075, 1083, 1089, 1090,
1091, 1092, 1093, 1102,
1103, 1104

Treefall
1017, 1018, 1045, 1068,
1075

*Variations on a Cellophane
Wrapper*
1006, 1007, 1008, 1010,
1011, 1012, 1015, 1017,
1018, 1021, 1026, 1027,
1028, 1037, 1041, 1043,
1045, 1051, 1052, 1054,
1056, 1061, 1063, 1066,
1068, 1071, 1072, 1074,
1075, 1083, 1103

Watching for the Queen
1034, 1035, 1045, 1050,
1051, 1052, 1057, 1058,
1064, 1067, 1068, 1071,
1075, 1082, 1083, 1089,
1090, 1092, 1093, 1103,
1106

West Coast
1010, 1011, 1012, 1017,
1018, 1022, 1045

Images on pages 3-4, 11-12, 15-16, 59-60, 95-96 are details of film stills from

Black Cat White Cat It's a Good Cat if It Catches the Mouse 1989

Graphic design: Bryan Gee

Printed in Canada

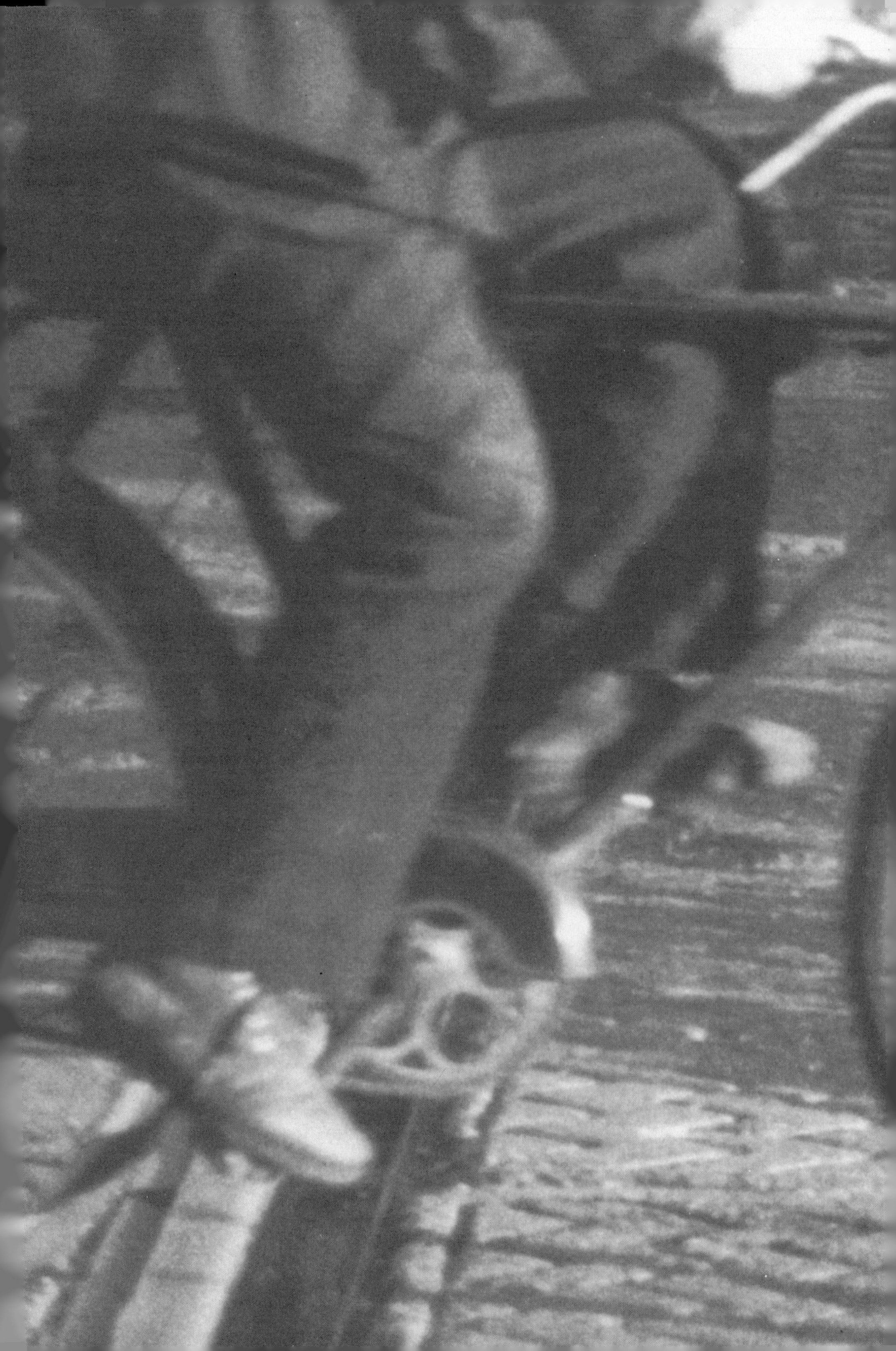

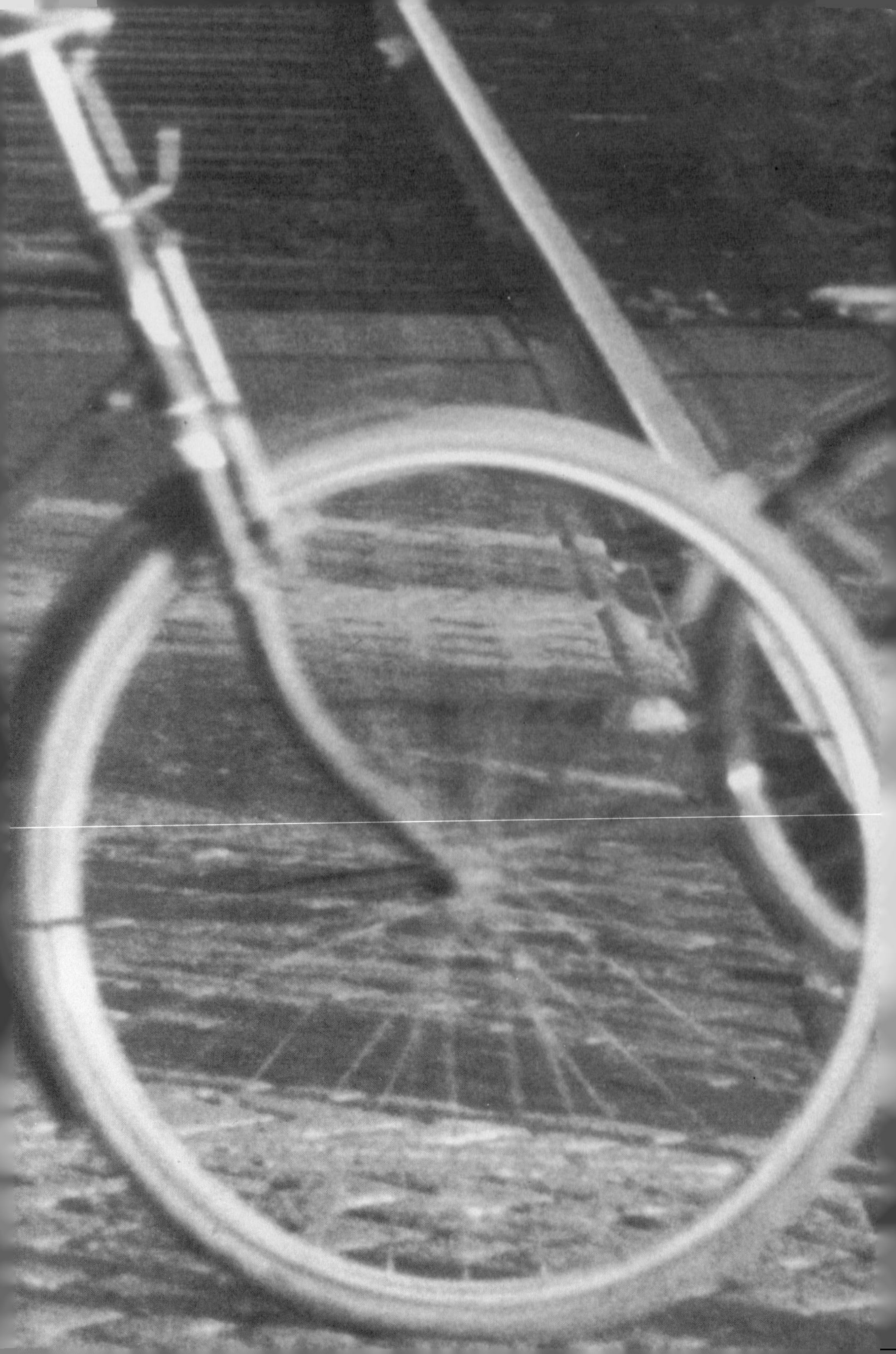